My Basketful of Happiness

"Why I Called Time on Alcohol"

Written By
Jonathan Dickin

First published in the United Kingdom in 2021
Self published by Jonathan Dickin

Cover design by Robert James Lee

Proof reading/Edited by Tiiu Shelley

"For my mate, Jeff. Thanks for the good times."
Andrew Dickin

My Dad, an Introduction

People have always told me that my Dad is "hilarious." As far back as I can remember, friends would tell me how funny my Dad is and that "it must be great to have a Dad as funny as him." I'd always disagree, of course, and tell them that he's a pain in the arse. From the second he wakes up in a morning until he crawls back into his "pit" at night, he's making bad jokes, or singing songs, or doing stupid voices… and usually, no matter what it is he does in his attempt to be amusing, he will look straight to me for a reaction, which is, more often than not, the thing that actually makes me laugh the most. But really, if I'm being completely honest, he is funny, and he really is a great Dad. He is largely responsible for shaping my tastes in music and comedy, he introduced me to some of my all-time favourite TV shows and movies (which largely consisted of watching The Office, Black Adder and Back To The Future day in, day out (sorry, Mum)), he took me to see bands in Manchester, Liverpool and Leeds (occasionally bands he'd never even heard of) and I can say with all sincerity that I wouldn't be the person I am today, for better or worse, without his influence.

There was one thing about my Dad, however, that influenced me more than anything else. His drinking habits. His influence in this particular field, however, was quite to the contrary of the aforementioned influences. "Everybody likes a drink", a nonsensical sound bite that gets spouted often, but there is nobody that that rings truer for than Andrew Dickin. As you'll read, my Dad's ambition was to be a drinker. As a young man, he actually idolised the people who could "hold their drink" and longed to earn that prestigious title for himself. It's safe to say, he did achieve that accolade and all that it entails. Some of my earliest memories of my Dad are of him with a pint glass in his hand, throwing the amber nectar down his gullet faster than I could drink my orange juice. And when the lager ran dry, out came the wine. Even to this day, at the ripe old age of 27, whenever I smell red wine, I picture my Dad draining the last drops of the bottle into his glass in order to pour on another. A nightly diet of lager and red wine went a long way towards creating the version of my Dad that I knew for the majority of my life thus far. It encompassed him in many ways, being the deciding factor in lots of his decision-making opportunities:

"Dad, can we go see this band on June 27th?"

"Yeah, no worries, what day is that on?"

"A Saturday"

"Oh, I can't be arsed with that"

Why? Because that meant driving, which meant not drinking on a weekend (he may have liked his drink, but he wouldn't risk his or our lives by drink driving). Heaven forbid he would take a night off from his drinking career. I must admit, in hindsight, there are some circumstances that came of his drinking that I'm thankful for. If he wasn't hungover on a weekend, maybe he'd have taken me to watch football matches, or even to football lessons. As a result of his drinking, this never happened, and I can proudly state that the Beautiful Game has no interest for me, so thanks, Dad.

Maybe this sounds as though I'm being a bit harsh on the man, after first stating that he's a great Dad and then going on to explain how we wouldn't do things together so he could fuel his addiction. But I know that's because the booze had him in its grasp, very, very tightly. I know it wasn't him making the decisions, it was the drink, or his "best friend" as he not so fondly refers to it these days. Obviously, as a kid, I didn't have any concept of this. I actually just assumed all Dads drank this much. That's what Dads do, surely! But as I got older and (much) wiser, I started to see my Dad's drinking problem as exactly that, a problem. I started to have an understanding of the damage this was doing. Four pint cans of Stella Artois and a bottle of Banrock Station a night isn't exactly cheap, and I don't just mean in terms of money. Weight gain, high blood pressure, strain on relationships, loss of a homegrown business, all of these stemmed from my Dad's best buddy and the choices he helped my Dad to make.

As you've no doubt surmised from my constant use of the past tense, my Dad is no longer a drinker. As of the time of writing this, he hasn't had a drop in 114 weeks. If you'd have told me 115 weeks ago that this would be the case, I would have laughed at you. He would tell us on a weekly basis (occasionally, nightly) that tonight was his "swan song", that he was definitely throwing in the towel after one more "party" - a party only ever had two people on the guest list, one of which was liquid based. I heard it that often that I actually grew tired of using the phrase "I'll believe it when I see it" when I was told he planned to say goodbye to his lifelong friend. *There's no way my Dad can give up drinking, the vice is so tight, it would take a miracle of will and determination to loosen it.* But I am immensely proud to say, he proved me and anybody else who doubted him wrong. With a resolve that I can only describe as miraculous, Andrew Dickin managed to cast off his alcohol-soaked life jacket and start a New Beginning. One that shocked and surprised not only me, but everyone who has ever known or cared for him.

My Dad first approached me about writing his story in 2019. He was just over a year into sobriety and was going through a phase of massive self-belief and confidence - which was rightly deserved, considering a year of sobriety was unheard of in the Andrew Dickin pantheon. It was during this time that he decided he wanted his story to be heard, no gory detail omitted. His belief was that there are many people the world over whose lives will have followed a similar trajectory to his own, leading them to believe that they couldn't and shouldn't quit drinking, that a liquid state is a fine future for themselves. He truly believes that the story of his transformation could serve as inspiration for many people to do the same but discussing his successes with people in passing can only go so far towards that goal. Naturally, he decided the best format for said story was a book. Once this idea came to him, that was it. A book *must* be written. There was just one problem standing in his way: Illiteracy.

Maybe that word is a bit strong; my Dad isn't technically illiterate. He can read and write to an extent that serves him adequately (he can text his friends about golfing and mountain biking, no problem), but he's never read a book from cover to cover in his life and his writing ability is poor at best. But he was under no false-pretense about this, hence why he asked me to be the medium for this story.

I suppose he decided I was most suited to write this book as I seem to be the most learned person in the family, being university educated (a degree in Music Production still counts as a degree, whether you like it or not) and being somewhat of a bookworm probably lead him to believe I understand books on a structural level. It's a common tradition in a "self-help" style book for the author to regale you with accomplishments, what qualifies them to impart their knowledge on you on a certain subject and why you should follow their lead. The most I can offer up in this regard is that I've written some music reviews on some online blogs, started and abandoned numerous writing projects and got a C at English GCSE. I make no claims to be an expert on the subject of alcohol, addiction or fitness and health, but before you decide to put this book down, remember that I have firsthand experience of what these things look like and what effects they can bring upon a person and the people around them. Me and my family have lived through addiction and that surely is worth something.

We talked at length about what structure this book should take and how it should be presented. The key word we struck upon early was "truth." This book will tell no lies or withhold any harsh realisations. It is simply the story of a man and the abusive relationship he had with his best friend. At times, you may think the tales within are funny (some of them are!), that my Dad enjoyed his time as a "piss head" and that's because he really believed that too, but that's beside the point. Every unit consumed just added to the problem until the penny dropped.

We're also conscious of the fact that not everybody wants to stop drinking. That's fine! This certainly isn't designed to be a preachy book and you won't find us calling alcohol "evil" or shaming people for their habits. But if you do feel that you have a problem and that your own experiences reflect that of my Dad's, or perhaps maybe you know someone who could use some guidance, our hope is that this book will serve as an eye opener as to the changes you can make in your life through determination and confidence.

When my Dad first christened the idea for this project, I admit to not believing he had the credentials to back it up. He was giddy with pride for what he had achieved up until that point, but there was a long journey ahead for him, one that he still proudly continues on with to this day. The idea wasn't written off entirely and stayed nestled in my Dad's mind, with the thought that when the time was right, he would ask me again. It just so happened, in 2020, the World became gripped in a pandemic of Biblical proportions, resulting in myself being out of work and with a lot of time on my hands, at which point, my Dad, now over 2 years sober, suggested once again that we collaborate to share his story. We had some "meetings" over some cups of Yorkshire's finest tea and the seeds were finally planted. The result - a story of a man and his relationship with alcohol: the ups, the downs, the beginnings, the endings. A story of one man and his basketful of happiness.

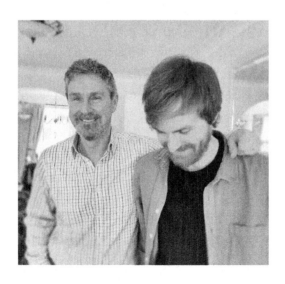

Chapter 1

Taming the Beast

We start this story at a time of disbelief and naivety from myself. There was nothing in my Dad's behaviour that I noticed in the time leading up to his decision to quit drinking to suggest to me, as someone who sees him daily, that such a cataclysmic change was coming to him. He spoke of quitting, but that was nothing new. For as long as he has identified with having a problem, he was "quitting", but it never materialised. He knew the issues existed, why else would he proclaim to be quitting so often? But his addiction persisted and won every mental war he waged within himself. My Dad would drink each and every night. But little did I or anyone else around him - I think even including him, himself - know that the next chapter of his life was about to be written right before our very eyes. As much as he wanted to believe it, he had burnt himself so many times in the past - as you shall discover in later chapters - only to turn back to his addiction worse than ever. But the shifting of the plates was fast approaching for my Dad, in the form of a storm, both physical and metaphorical. To fully appreciate the drastic change this meant for my Dad, a wealth of back story is required, to understand just how much his addiction affected every facet of his life. But what is more fascinating and illuminating is the betterment of his life following this shift.

So, we start at the turning point, the shifting of the scales, when he discarded the hand he had chosen for himself, to be dealt the unknown, the terrifying and yet the greatest hand he could have hoped for.

. . . .

Saturday, Feb 24th, 2018 - A particularly exciting day for Andrew, or for all of us in actual fact, as our friends, the Bates, were paying us a visit and staying over for the night. It's a friendship that goes back to childhood. Andrew's wife, Christine (who will make many appearances throughout), has been best friends with the mother of the family, Ingrid, as far back as primary school. That friendship has remained a very large part of Andrew and Christine's life right up to present day and also resulted in the friendship of Andrew and Jeff, Ingrid's husband. In the early days, the two couples would often do things as a foursome, double-dating, if you will. The friendship between all parties grew stronger through this time of blossoming romantic relationships, with Christine and Ingrid being thrilled to find that their sweethearts could also become such close friends. But, unfortunately, there was a third wheeler tagging along at most gatherings. Mr Cohol. Al, Cohol.

As much as Andrew enjoys the time spent with these wonderful people, as most events in his life did, such visits and occasions would serve as the perfect opportunity to become better acquainted with Al. His destructive consumption was expanded to new levels when with Jeff, as he would join Andrew in drinking to excess. Things got so out of hand on numerous occasions that Christine and Ingrid actually stopped seeing each other as much, perhaps subconsciously, both aware that the evenings would always end in the same way. I suppose you could call it "damage control." Trying to somehow limit or maintain the situation.

Ingrid and Jeff, along with their young children, made the decision to move from the surrounding area, following Jeff obtaining a new job. With a two-and-a-half-hour drive now separating them, Andrew and Jeff's wild nights seemed like a thing of the past. But the friendship maintained throughout the years and gatherings would be arranged on a semi-regular basis, with either us (us now consisting of Andrew, Christine, my older brother Chris and myself) going to stay with them or for them (them now consisting of Ingrid, Jeff, Dominic, Angharad and Christian) to come stay with us.

And so, back to the story, this particular Saturday was an exciting one, as the Bates' were en route. I have many happy memories of these weekends. Christine would be thrilled to get to spend the night in the company of her best friend, myself and Dominic would get to spend the night discussing Pokemon cards and Video games (we took these things very seriously, to the point of being dubbed "The Philosophers" by Jeff), we would all get to enjoy a banquet of a Chinese take away and Andrew and Jeff would get to open a can or two. And a bottle or two. And then another can or two. And on the night would flow, a river of amber, red and intoxication.

The evening in question was attended only by Christine, Andrew, Ingrid, Jeff and Christian, as us older ones either didn't live at home anymore, were out with our own partners or simply had prior engagements. However, despite this change to the attendance, one element of the night maintained the status quo of previous visits; Andrew had consumed far too much alcohol and was sprawled out, fast asleep on the living room floor, shirt ridden up to reveal his stomach, which had grown exponentially over the years, and snoring like a jet engine. A beached whale comes to mind. Jeff, on the other hand, would still be wide awake and would be sat with the rest of the party, watching television (turned up loud enough to drown out Free Willy at their feet) and joining in the conversation. Yes, he joined Andrew in drinking on these nights, but he wouldn't let himself get into a similar state, pumping the brakes slightly if things started accelerating too quickly, where Andrew would accelerate more rapidly with each drink consumed. He would eventually wake up some time in the early hours of the morning, bewildered and bleary eyed and stumble his way up the stairs and collapse into bed.

Always the early bird, whatever state he may be in, he would be up before anyone else, downstairs making a coffee. Maybe this was an attempt to assert himself as "right as rain" before the rest of the house would wake up and see the man who resembled a large, helpless, aquatic mammal 8 hours prior. As the kettle boiled, Ingrid joined him in the kitchen. "Morning, Andrew", she said in the ever so friendly way she does.

"Morning, Little Thing", he responded. The charade began, as he attempted to disguise the adverse effects the previous night's debauchery had left residing within him, masked by politeness and apparent normality.

"How are you feeling this morning?" Ingrid chuckled.

"Oh, I'm right as rain" he'd continue the deception. This sort of aftermath normalcy was nothing out of the ordinary, but Andrew recalls feeling particularly embarrassed at this point, as he stood close to Ingrid in the Kitchen. *"She must think I look like a horrendous, bloated mess"*, he thought to himself, as the lingering smell of red wine clung to him like a well-worn cloak. The morning would unfold as usual, with the rest of the house slowly waking up, the smell of bacon crisping under the grill, the kettle being put through its paces and the whole crew gathering in the living room to have the first conversation of the weekend of which alcohol wasn't a part, all the while Andrew continued to feel worse for wear.

Around lunch time, old friends would bid each other farewell, and the customary "night after the party" blues would set in for both Christine and Andrew. The former would then begin operation clean up to try and bring back some composure to the house while latter would continue to feel lethargic and useless, watching some football highlights from the sofa. As is tradition on most Sunday's, my parents would make plans to visit

Christine's father and stepmother, Adrian and Margaret, who live a short walk away, a couple of streets over, a tradition that goes back to the start of their relationship.

Visiting his father-in-law is something Andrew has always enjoyed. He thoroughly relishes the company of Adrian and Margaret, who would no doubt have him laughing very soon upon entering the house and so visiting them never felt a chore, as it is often presented by fictional families. Sometimes, particularly in the early days, they may play a card game or two. Sometimes, they may find themselves sitting in the summer house at the back of the garden, weather permitting. But, always, Adrian would say the magic words. Similar in effect to that immortal phrase imparted upon us by Ali Baba, he would say, "go and help yourself to a beer, Andrew."

"Are you sure?" came his response, the customary politeness, already beginning his journey to the fridge.

"Of course, get me one while you're there" replied Adrian. Ahh, the hair of the dog. The one single, sure-fire way to cure a hangover, according to nearly all drinkers the world over. The theory states that consuming more alcohol while in a hungover state will actually quell the illness and get you back on your feet, presumably ready to consume ever more. And so the vicious circle continues, regulating your body to a state of alcohol familiarity. A hangover sets in when your blood alcohol level reaches zero. In other words, the alcohol consumed the day before has now left your bloodstream. Your body doesn't know how to process this and so severe sickness symptoms start to show. Headaches, nausea, lack of appetite and more. It can often result in the ejection of bodily fluids via the mouth. Or elsewhere. However, by consuming more alcohol while in this self-afflicted state, the blood alcohol level increases again and the body receives what it has been conditioned to crave. Hey presto, no more hangover. That is, of course, until the level reaches zero again in a matter of hours, and the process can start once more. I suppose the hair of the dog can almost be viewed as a training regime for alcoholics. Keep up the training for a while and you'll be a fully-fledged drinker before you know it! And so, of course, for a well-practiced guzzler such as Andrew, this method is well ingrained.

With that, we return to the opening of Sesame, better known as Grandad Adrian's fridge. What treasures would be held within today? Some Belgian beer? Maybe some cans of Asahi from Japan? But what's wrong with a good old Stella Artois? In truth, it didn't matter, so long as it was cold, golden and primed to enter Andrew's system. A couple of cans in hand, Andrew returned to the cosy back room, with the fire roaring and the conversation flowing. Over the course of the next hour or so, he would make three more trips to the fridge, bringing the total amount of dog hairs to four. It's at this point that Mr Cohol appears to talk exclusively to Andrew. He whispers into his ear, "why stop there?" Andrew agrees and so upon leaving, he insists that Christine drive him to the petrol station at the bottom of the hill, Andrew's favoured purveyor of beverages and a place he visits on a daily basis, where he picks up another four pint cans of Stella and a bottle of red wine, the standard, nightly medication. Like a greedy child with a bag of sweets, he can't wait to get stuck in. Back into his favoured spot on the sofa, pint glass in hand, wine warming near the radiator.

But it's at this point that something changes. It could hardly be described as miraculous, after all, he'd already drunk his fair share for the night, but Andrew only drank one of the cans. Admittedly, he drank all the wine, yes, but he left three pint cans of Stella in the fridge and called it a night (by which I mean he fell asleep on the sofa, once again). What seems like little room for celebration could also be seen as the first step towards Andrew walking away from his lifelong friend. The following morning,

Andrew wakes up in a very similar state to the day before. Blood alcohol at zero and feeling worse for wear, his favoured cape once again draped over him. He turns to Christine and says, "never again", a personal creed, one I think he never truly believed in himself, but I suppose it imbues a feeling of defiance, if only temporarily. He tells her that's it. No more. Finito. Sayonara, Al. Although she'd truly like to believe him this time, the words fall on deaf ears, as Christine has heard this an unfathomable amount of times.

Andrew left for work as usual. Following in his father's footsteps, Andrew is a painter and decorator and often works with my brother, Chris, his eldest son, who has continued the tradition of learning the trade from *his* Dad. That Monday, they were working in Yockenthwaite, North Yorkshire, with Matt Heap, a personal friend of ours. On the way to work, the big news on the radio was "The Beast from the East", the cold wave that was due to sweep across the United Kingdom. Although it *officially* began on February 22nd, our area wouldn't be affected by it until a few days later. But already, news reports were coming in of huge amounts of snow and generally disruptive weather in parts of the UK. At work, Chris was excitedly talking about the storm, like a kid listening to the local radio in hopes that they'll inform him school is closed tomorrow. "We're apparently going to get five foot of snow!" Chris announces, with more than a little hope in his voice.

After work, Andrew arrived home to an empty house, as Christine was out for a birthday meal for her stepfather, Robert. She'd left him some food to prepare for himself and said she wouldn't be back too late. Andrew put his tea in the oven, took off his overalls and got ready to settle into a relaxing evening after work. As he moved through the house, he heard a voice and it sounded trapped. "Dri...... e....." the voice sounds muffled, but after a short search, he narrows it down to the fridge. He approaches it with some trepidation and slowly pulls open the fridge door to find Al sat on the shelf in the form of the three pint cans of Stella he neglected the night before. "Drink me!", he yells at Andrew. As he reaches out to take him in his hand, he thinks "but I told Christine this morning I was done." He looks back to Al and that thought quickly subsides, as Al deceptively plants a new one there. "Ah well, might as well as finish these off and then I can start again tomorrow." And with that, all notion of today being the end is out the window. He pours the first can into an official Stella Artois pint glass (such a big fan he even has the official merchandise. And not the knocked off stuff sold by the dodgy bloke outside after the show, the real deal!) and begins to gulp away. He takes his tea out of the oven and seats himself at the breakfast bar, where he proceeds to nail all three cans in a short span of time.

Christine arrives home from the meal while he is sat in the Kitchen and notices a cheeky smile plastered across his face. "What's up?" she asks suspiciously.

"Nothing", he replies with a small laugh, knowing he has done wrong, but trying to pass it off as a bit of a joke. She sees the empty cans by the garage door and the oh too familiar notion of "so all that you said about never again?" is present once more. "Yeah, well I thought I might as well finish what was in the house and then I'll start properly from tomorrow." *Yeah, ok Andrew, whatever.*

Tuesday, Feb 27th, 2018 - Overnight, Chris's prayers were answered. The North West of the UK met with the full force of "The Beast from the East." All across the area, people were waking up and looking out onto the thick blanket of snow that had transformed the area into that wondrous place Dean Martin used to sing about. Kids across the area would share Chris's excitement at the prospect of a snow day, the news would report that local services had been heavily affected by the weather and early risers would be out enjoying the wonderful crisp satisfaction of freshly laid snow underfoot as they took that morning stroll. Andrew, however, was about to awaken, in more ways than one. He opened his eyes and was greeted once again by a hangover. But, as he recalls, this wasn't like any ordinary hangover. In his words, he felt a new degree of illness, as though he had transcended the usual state of withdrawal, to one that left him feeling like he had done irreparable damage to himself. For a man as stubborn in his defiance as Andrew, to admit to such weakness was rare. As someone who has experienced some level of hangover daily for the majority of his adult life, he knew this was different. For some reason, those last three golden bullets the night before had planted themselves deeply.

While retelling this story today, Andrew actually starts to feel the sickness he felt that morning. Such a powerful hangover that it carries residual pain with it, even to this day, over two years later.

He sits himself up in bed and reaches for a small pocket diary on his bedside table, rarely used. Ironically, the diary was branded with a Brewery logo. He turns to today's date and writes two simple words. Two words that probably didn't mean all that much at the time, but would go on to be the next chapter of his life. In fact, this was greater than a chapter break. This was more like the start of Season 2. Or the hugely successful sequel to a rather lackluster movie. Andrew Dickin 2. But I digress. The two simple words…

Spelling mistake and all, Andrew had made his stand. And this time, it was in writing.

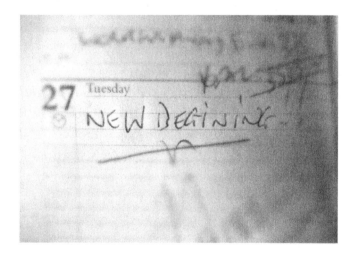

As he sat on the side of his bed with his feet on the ground, a great amount of fear and anxiety washed over him. Rather like the ice bucket challenge craze from a few years ago, where participants would make exclamations of fear, knowing the contents of the bucket about to be poured over them would be intensely cold, but unaware of the extent of that coldness. The difference in this case was that this bucket of alcohol-induced dread was being poured by Al himself. He was saying, "oh yeah? You think you can break up with me that easily? How about some of this?" Holidays, Christmas, nights with friends, visits from the Bates, Grandad Adrian, birthdays, family gatherings… what would any of these be like without Al by his side, or, more accurately, in his blood? Throughout his whole life since the age of 18, all of these events and more have been fueled by drink. They were inconceivable without it and it actually frightened my Dad. How could he possibly sit in a beautiful restaurant in Majorca, with a breathtaking view of the sunset at sea, the love of his life by his side, the best food money can buy in front of him and not throw back some cold, refreshing beer and wash it down with a lovely drop of red? It was inconceivable for him and genuinely terrifying. He knew there and then that this would be the single most difficult process of his life. The fear of the unknown could easily have been enough to see an end to this hangover induced decision before it has even been put into action.

Fear wouldn't be the only hurdle on this path; there are numerous trials and tribulations that come with making a decision like this, impatience being another example. It's a very cruel thing, impatience, when you think about it. When you really set your mind to obtaining a goal, whether that be to lose weight, gain muscle, learn an instrument, write a book, whatever it is you strive for, what you're really saying is, "I want that", as in, you want to be at that end goal straight away. You want to be that target weight, you want to be able to bench press that much, you want to be able to play Mozart's Symphony No. 40 blindfolded. Andrew is no stranger to being impatient. In fact, I've often described him as being the most impatient man I've ever met. And so, by committing to this "New Beginning", he had to be at the end goal straight away. There was no weaning off drink. With an oft utilised all or nothing attitude, that was to be the end of it. So, without wasting another minute, he commandeered Christine's iPad, opened YouTube and searched for "quit drinking." He quickly hit upon some videos by a man called Craig Beck. Craig has a YouTube channel devoted entirely to motivational videos on how to give up alcohol, having once been an alcoholic himself. He has become very successful through his videos and books, in which he shares his pathways to success when dealing with addiction. With the weather outside growing increasingly worse, Andrew laid back in bed and watched a few of said videos. After a while, he came downstairs and excitedly told Christine about what he had found, telling her that he really thinks this guy knows the secret to giving up. They did a little research and found that Craig had released a book entitled "Alcohol Lied to Me." Now, as you've previously learnt, as much as he'd really love to, Andrew can't read a book. Never in his life has he managed to read one from start to finish. However, thanks to the wonderful, ever growing power of the internet, there was an audiobook option available. The stars aligned, as Christine had a credit available to download one audiobook, which she kindly donated to Andrew - of course, she would be willing to try anything to help him succeed in his mission. And so, with his book downloaded, he went back to bed and spent the best part of the day fully engrossed in Craig's story, one that reflected his own in so many ways.

Over the course of a week, one which continued to see the UK battered by the proverbial beast, which, naturally had Brits reacting in that oh so British way - absolutely everything shut down, this is the next ice age, blah blah blah - Andrew stayed inside and continued to listen to the inspiring words of Craig Beck. It became a morning ritual for him: wake up, make brew, go back to bed, listen to audiobook, commence day feeling ready to face the inevitable cravings of a person giving up their cherished love. The first week is, quite naturally, in most cases, the most difficult time for somebody giving up an addiction. They call it "drying out" or going "cold turkey." A person who has become so reliant on a substance will experience huge withdrawal symptoms during this phase, while the body tries to formulate new coping methods now that a key functionality ingredient is missing. Having tried (and failed) to give up booze before, this phase was no stranger to Andrew, but he recalls that this time, it felt way more intense than previous efforts; Al really didn't want to let go of my Dad's hand. The fierce hangover he experienced on the 27th lingered for the entire week, as though the snow flurries outside carried within them the source of his anguish. As they continued to blow, he continued to suffer. He claims to have only ever experienced a hangover of this magnitude once before in his life - don't forget, he would normally extinguish the fire with beer, an option no longer available to him, if he is to commit to his life altering decision. And so the temptation to relapse was already huge for him, even just a few days into this journey. In his own words: "I'd wake up every day that week and think "what is going on?" I didn't understand how I could still be feeling that ill. It just wouldn't go away." However, unperturbed, he continued with Craig's book, following his instructions to the letter. At one point, the book mentioned some vitamins and supplements that help fight the cravings and so, without a moment wasted, Andrew ventured out into the storm to the chemists to get everything Craig told him to.

Something else recommended by the book was to work out just how much money was being spent on alcohol on an annual basis. This was a huge factor in Andrew's decision to quit. In fact, he would argue it was the first and foremost reason to do so. We have never been a particularly *"well off"* family. We have mostly always had enough to live comfortably (speaking from my perspective, at least for as long as I can remember) and there are certainly innumerable amounts of people worse off financially than us, but we hit upon hard ground a few years ago, where we faced possible eviction from our home. They were dark days, exaggerated by Andrew's incessant, daily spending on his fuel. Following Craig's advice, my Dad worked out his daily alcohol expenditure, then his weekly, then his monthly and eventually, his yearly. It shocked him to discover that he was spending nearly £4,000 a year on drinking. Not only that, but his monthly outgoings on drink were exceeding that of the mortgage repayments. He was drinking our family's finances into oblivion, while only just affording to keep the roof over our heads. When you think about what that actually represents, the fact that he was spending a very large amount of money on urinating and feeling ill, it really is very alarming and was the spark that lit the flame underneath Andrew. This was a truly eye opening realisation for him.

A storm from the Russian Far East, a chance encounter with an audiobook, support from friends and family and an unbreakable will had laid the foundations of what would be the next stage of Andrew's life. It would be an incredibly difficult path to follow, with a tremendous amount of temptation, doubt, fear, anxiety and just about every other negative connotation primed to make an appearance along the way. And with that rocky and tumultuous road laid out ahead, let's now go backwards, to explore the root of the addiction, the defining moments of Andrew's life with his illness, the incredible lows experienced - alongside the undeniable high moments - and the eventual desire to make huge changes in his life.

Chapter 2

I Want to Drink & Drive

When I first started to write this book, I found I argued with myself as to what the actual aim of the book was; is it a true story of a man battling with addiction, told in a novel-esque way? Is it a self-help book designed to inspire people to quit drinking? Is it simply the translation of one man's story via his son, who witnessed a lot of it? Is it supposed to be humorous and relatable, or is it supposed to be alarming and eye-opening? I quickly realised it could be all those things.

I wanted to be able to tell my Dad's story in a way that people would find humorous and endearing, but also in the hopes that people could maybe see themselves, or someone they care about, and then possibly they might say, "wow, this sounds familiar. If he can do it, so can I."

. . . .

Andrew tells me that when he was younger, he had two ambitions for his future: Drink and Drive. I was relieved when he went on to tell me that he didn't mean simultaneously. He has always imbued an incredible passion for wanting to be the best at everything he did. Even to this day, whenever he latches on to a new hobby, he has to be the best at it straight away. Mountain biking: after riding for a month or two, already tackling huge rides. Golfing: swings a club once, needs all the best gear and goes for a round nightly. Thankfully, this quality of him I believe also helped his passion towards quitting drinking. But as a teenager, he had different aims.

Andrew grew up in a small village in Lancashire called Kelbrook. A very quiet place to spend his formative years, with a small, tight community where everybody knows everybody, and most people are farmers and wear flat caps. Think Last of the Summer Wine and you're probably along the right tracks. He lived there with his Mum and Dad, Shirley and George (my wonderful grandparents) and his older sister, Kath. He had a fantastic upbringing in this setting, seeing his Dad work very hard as a painter and decorator (who would go on to take Andrew on as his apprentice and teach him the ways of the brush) and had many friends that he spent most of his waking hours with, playing in the surrounding moors, fishing for bullheads and beck jumping. An idyllic upbringing, in many regards. From a young age, Andrew was someone who would go through hobbies like socks and, each time he discovered a new one, he would become addicted to it and would strive for perfection. He would soon move on to something else and become just as enamoured with that. He became known to some in the village as "Gonna Dickin", as in, "what's he gonna be into next?" This addictive personality was quite possibly a precursor to what would come later in his life but was seen as little more than a young man who wanted to try everything and be the best at it all. Jack of all and all that.

At age 14, Andrew developed an insatiable desire to drive. He would fantasise about being old enough to start taking driving lessons and longed for the freedom of having his own car and being able to go anywhere and do anything he wanted. He wanted this so badly, he would quite literally wish his time away, pleading to be 17 so he could get his provisional and scratch this unrelenting motor-based itch. Perhaps it came from spending so much time with his best friend, Richard Wilson, who lived on a farm. Driving the tractors, seeing the 4X4's and anything else with an engine must have got under his skin and driven (pardon the pun) his desire forward.

1982 rolled around and Andrew turned 17. He got his provisional driving licence as soon as humanly possible and got booked in for his very first driving lesson. With his determination to be the best operating at full capacity, Andrew learned incredibly quickly. He was quite simply a natural. At the end of his first lesson, his driving instructor said, "well, let's get you booked in for your test." He was beside himself, well on his way to achieving his goal of being a driver, and most likely the first of his friend group in the village - hence, the best. He took three more lessons before the day of his test arrived, during which he continued to impress his instructor. Naturally, he passed his test first try and he was there. Goal achieved. Andrew Dickin, driving extraordinaire at age 17. With that out of the way, he needed a new goal. One that he could pour just as much passion into and really focus all his energy on. But with such a wide world of opportunities out there, what was he "gonna" do next? A lot of people would maybe delve into books to find inspiration, or television, documentaries, movies, whatever it may be. Andrew, however, found his inspiration in Kelbrook's local watering hole, the Craven Heifer.

The Heifer, as it's known locally, was everything you imagine a village pub to be. Kelbrook's farming community would meet there of an evening and discuss cows and grass and whatever it is farmers talk about (they have their own language, so it could be anything), darts would fly across the room and the smell of beer, cigarettes and cow shit would fill the air. Picturesque. Dennis Murray was the landlord at the time. Being a local, close-knit community, Dennis would let youngsters into the pub to drink cola and play card games and relax, usually under the supervision of their fathers, who would no doubt be propping the bar up and sipping on an ale. However, he would under no circumstances allow underage drinking. Instead, he offered a free shot of rum to people on their 18th birthday. Welcome to the big leagues, sort of thing.

Andrew's Dad, George, was a regular at the Heifer. He would go there frequently to see friends and drink "Mild" beer (if you're not sure what mild beer is, imagine a nice cold mug of muddy puddle). Occasionally, Andrew would join his Dad, along with a few friends, who would spend the evening drinking soft drinks. It was during this time of youthful innocence that Andrew started to develop an admiration for the men at the bar. More specifically, for their drinking habits. He started to understand the difference between those who could "hold" their drink and those who didn't quite have that knack. He started to view it as a form of accomplishment. The folk who could drink pint after pint and stay firmly planted on the tap room floor became heroes in his eyes, like top scoring football players or platinum selling recording artists. These men held just as much esteem for Andrew as any of those. Truly, kings among men. And they were! They were some of the nicest chaps you could ever ask to meet, as these sorts of quiet ale houses bred that type of person. Ok, so they might look at you funny when you walk in for the first time as a newcomer, but that's only because they didn't recognise you, and that was alien to them in a village like Kelbrook. It wouldn't take long for a stranger to be ingratiated into the pack. But Andrew saw his destiny in these men. The ability to hold one's own, he longed for. It became his next goal. This was what Andrew was "gonna" do next: Drink.

And so there he was, 17 years old and counting down the days until Dennis would grant him that oh so longed after shot of brown, foul liquid. Much like his ambition to drive, except where his driving lessons opened up the possibility to travel far and wide, the lessons he undertook for this test only required one single destination - the Heifer - and he went there as often as possible to learn the ways of the ale. As he sat there and admired the locals, a man approached him who he didn't recognise. He took a seat next to Andrew, leaned forward and said, "don't worry, son. It won't be long now. We're going to have such a great time together, you and me. You've still got a lot to learn, but I can tell we're going to be close." He would later come to recognise this man as his close friend. Andrew, at this time, didn't quite comprehend what a friendship with this character could possibly mean for his future. All that mattered right now was getting that rum down his neck!

Andrew would often visit the pub with his cousin and close friend Steven. S Man to those who know him. Whether S Man had the same desire to experience alcohol as Andrew did, I'm not sure, but they were certainly together the first time Steven would get his initial taste. It was his 18th birthday and so, naturally, there was only one thing for it: to the Heifer! Andrew was green with envy. S Man was going to get the rum that he so desired. And it wasn't even nearly his birthday yet! The wait would go on, the days slowly ticking by. They opened the door and took a step inside, greeted by the usual sights and smells and made their way up to the bar. Dennis approached them at the bar, knowing it was S Man's big day - his purification ceremony - time to ingratiate him. "Right then young man, it's your turn." He turns and grabs the bottle, pulls out the stopper and pours out one shot of the cherished spirit, places it in front of him on the bar. Everyone in the pub was looking on, a few expectant laughs emerging from them, knowing full well that the reaction will be a sour one. S Man looks round, like he's ready to perform on stage to a large crowd of adoring fans. He takes one last look at my Dad, lifts the shot glass to his lips and tips his head backwards. He swallows, puts the glass back on the bar, looks round at the waiting audience and eloquently announces "that tastes like badger piss", which sends Andrew into fits of laughter and leaves the rest of the pub in silence. But though S Man's reaction was hilarious to him, the real feeling was jealousy. *S Man is there now*, he thought. *He's done it, he's arrived*. He can drink now, what a thing to be envious of.

Time slowly trickled by, Andrew still desperate for that first taste of "manhood." Trips to the Heifer had changed, somewhat. They were still the same in most regards, but now S Man would have a pint or two, while Andrew still sat there sipping away at his cola. It only made the wait more difficult as he sat and imagined the day he'd be chucking down pint after pint, with people admiringly saying "wow, he can really drink."

Finally, the big day came. Andrew turned 18. A big day in anybody's life. It feels like a huge turning point for so many people. Although most will continue to act like children for many years to come - as of the time of writing, Andrew is 54, and I'm still not sure if maturity ever really came to him - this is the first foray into adulthood. The early maturers would be planning the next stage of their lives, falling in love, looking for work - whatever it may be - but Andrew still had unfinished business to attend to before any of that took priority. He couldn't mature into adulthood without first experiencing this long dreamt of moment. He stepped out of his front door, walked 50 yards, rounded the corner and there she stood. The venue for this most auspicious ceremony, the scene of his ascension into manhood - The Craven Heifer.

As had been the case with S Man a year earlier, he opened the doors and stepped inside, approached the bar and awaited Dennis's pouring of the rum. The stopper came out, the shot glass went down. It was time. He picked up his glass and took one last look around the room. He noticed a man sat at the end of the bar. He'd seen him before, but he couldn't quite remember where. Re-focusing on the important stuff, he raised up the shot glass and poured it in. It's funny, but at that moment, destiny, as it turned out, tasted awful. It was much stronger than he had anticipated and not particularly enjoyable and he agreed that it definitely resembled the urine of some form of weasel. But it didn't matter. He'd done it. He returned the shot glass to the bar and was patted on the back by the mysterious man from the end of the bar, who shook his hand and said, "hi, I'm Al." He spent the rest of the evening in his company, as he enjoyed his first taste of manhood, and what better way to prove his manhood than to drink what the men drank, mild beer - when in Rome, I suppose.

To refer back to Andrew's passion to drive, we can consider this series of events to be the first lesson in his drinking education. Of course, it was too soon for people to start to refer to him as a "drinker", or someone who can "hold their drink", but he'd learnt the fundamentals: The taste, the sensation, the cost (roughly 70p a pint) and most importantly, he'd become acquainted with his instructor/new buddy, Al. The next step would be to refine his skills and prove to people that he could achieve his goal and that he could do it quickly. That meant getting his name out there, being seen with a pint glass in his hand. Kelbrook was solid ground for the first lesson, a good way to get his feet wet, but if he was to prove himself, he was going to have to spread his wings a little and get out there. The nearest town to Kelbrook would be Earby, a small town only a couple of miles up the road. Andrew would set off on a Friday night headed for the Brummel, one of Earby's finest drinking establishments, which happened to be situated right at the far end of town. He would walk straight past the bus stop, pocketing what would have been bus money for the sole purpose of being able to buy another pint or two with it. Real commitment. Occasionally, he would make the journey with friends with whom he would spend the evening with, or he'd bump into people he knew at the Brummel. But if not, it didn't matter. He'd make the trip either way and if he was on his own, sat at the bar throwing beers down, then so be it. Having nobody by his side wasn't going to interrupt his strenuous training programme. And in all honesty, this probably strengthened his image as a boozer. Only a true boozer, someone who really loved the stuff, would sit there and do it on their own, even at the age of 18. Al was always there, though. He'd never let him down. Such a dependent and loyal friend.

Andrew was lucky in his drinking in that the early days didn't come with hangovers, or at least not to the extent that the later days would. There is very little science backing this up, but most people who have experienced hangovers throughout their life will tell you that symptoms grow in severity with age. This is likely due to the fact that we lose muscle and gain fat, the older we get, in most cases. Muscle is composed of a significantly lower percentage of water than fat and with alcohol being absorbed by water content within the body, the higher the body fat amount, the more alcohol absorbed and the longer it will stay in the system. With Andrew being a sporty, fit young man at this point in his life, the day after hardly seemed a hurdle. So, what may have seemed a deterrent, in the form of negative side effects, didn't really occur. And if there *was* some lingering after party downers, Al would simply get in touch with his bag of magic dog hairs, the ultimate medicine. And so it seemed that Andrew could only see the good side of drinking. The buzz of being drunk, the ever-growing image, the laughs. In fact, he only recalls one negative from those days (aside from the later realisation of being on a one-way tramline it would be difficult to get off) and that was anxiety over his actions while intoxicated. He wouldn't have thought of it as anxiety at the time, not wanting to take anything away from the macho image, and with mental health not really being a global concern at the time and people bottling up emotions a lot more for fear of being labeled "mad" or "crazy." But he recalls feeling a certain degree of concern over things he had said to people the night before. He remembered with absolute clarity *what* he had said, but with his inhibitions lowered by the alcohol fueling him the night before, he would often say things he would regret the day after. This anxiety could have tripped up his progress, could have possibly been a stumbling block or a cap on things, but instead, Al imparted more wisdom upon him.

He learned to say, "ah fuck it, I'll just buy them a drink next time I see them, be reyt." And so booze was the answer, as it would be for many future issues. Another lesson in the bag for this blossoming drinker.

A few months into his rigorous training schedule, Andrew and his friends booked a holiday to Spain. A "lads" holiday. A perfect opportunity for him to put his lessons in to practice and to show Spain what a world class drinker he could be. A true legend. El Dickin. Along with his pals, Anthony and Nigel, he got the coach across the channel. Maybe it was the excitement of what was to come (giddiness being something Andrew has maintained to this day), he got stuck into the booze straight away and ended up throwing up on the coach. But with his mates having his back, the mishap was quickly laughed off. Something which is referred to these days as "tactical chundering." Getting that up to put more drink down. Lovely. It certainly didn't dampen his spirits as he cracked open another can with the lads and continued on his escapade.

Upon arriving, they met up with their friends Nibs and Bodger, who were already there to start the party early. The five of them were there for two weeks, staying in a full board hotel. Wasting no time, they hit the bars, getting a feel for their favourites, sampling the beer on offer and discovering a love for drinking Bacardi and Coke, perfect for the Spanish climate. It seemed ideal, to Andrew. This was everything he had hoped for in drinking. It delivered massively. He was having a great time with his friends, laughing endlessly, smoking Spain's finest 'Fortuna' cigarettes (Andrew wasn't really much of a smoker, but it helped strengthen his image further, because all men smoke, *obviously*) and draining the land of its supply of Bacardi. They weren't there to cause trouble or be unruly, they weren't even there to try and "pull" girls, or at least Andrew wasn't. It was just a chance for him and his friends to experience what the world of booze had to offer outside Kelbrook and Earby.

Andrew quickly discovered a favourite drinking establishment by the name of 'The Flying Horse'. Whatever the others were up to, he would always end up making his way there and drinking with the regulars, who came to know him and saw him as something of a "legend." Dad's dreams were coming true! He was that determined to drink, that he would actually abandon his dinner halfway through and head to the Horse. Eating only meant getting full, leaving less room for drink. So he'd stand up from the table and tell his friends where they could find him, like they needed telling.

One night, Nigel decided to speak up. Andrew did his usual, got bored of his meal halfway through, pushed his chair back when Nigel said, "I'm coming with you. I'm going to keep up with you tonight." The rest of them tried to tell Nigel that probably wouldn't be a good idea. Andrew's ego inflated. They saw him as someone it would be hard to keep up with! The training was paying off after all!

"Come on then, let's go to The Flying Horse", Andrew replied. In they walk, a Fortuna burning away between his fingers. "two Bacardi and Cokes please." And so they started Andrew's nightly routine, puffing and guzzling away. But things quickly ended for Nigel "Nanny" Francis, as they used to call him. The booze was too much for him and too quick. He ended up stumbling his way back to the hotel, where he happened to be sharing a room with Andrew. Andrew went and found the others and they headed up to their room where they found Nanny had locked himself in the bathroom. They could hear ungodly gurgling noises from behind the door as Nanny ejected all that he had thrown down his neck. Naturally, they all found this highly amusing, but started to grow concerned as each minute rolled by without so much as a glimpse of Nanny, still getting better acquainted with the porcelain bowl inside. The noise had ceased, but the door remained locked. "Nanny, open the door, mate" they shouted as they banged on, hoping to keep him at least conscious. Just as panic started to really set in, the lock turned and out came Nanny, "looking like a zombie" as he stumbled out of the door and collapsed on to his bed. He was absolutely trollied. They all laughed and joked and Andrew stood proud, having drunk just as much, if not more, and feeling like an absolute hero to his friends. "My God, look what trying to keep up with Andrew has done to Nanny. You're my hero Andrew, you really can drink!" is probably what he would have liked one of them to say at that stage, but the fantasy will have to make do.

For the rest of the holiday, Andrew and Nibs spent most of their time together, as he was pretty much the only one who could keep up. They would continue to frequent the Horse, drinking and smoking enough for the rest of the party. Again, the hangovers didn't set in for these young men. The only experience was the buzz. They were so thrilled to be doing exactly as they were.

The holiday did as all good things must - it ended. Two weeks of living the dream came to a close as they all boarded the coach and headed back to that loveliest of villages, Kelbrook. But it wasn't quite enough for Andrew, it never is. So the day he arrived home, he saw his parents and his sister, threw his luggage down, quickly changed his clothes and headed straight for Earby. The Brummel was waiting. So the party rolled on for Andrew, once again. After all, he's a drinker now, just ask Nanny, if he's recovered. He took his place at the bar and resumed his training, same as ever. Except he noticed things were different. The atmosphere had changed somehow. Maybe it was due to having such a good time with his friends or the camaraderie he experienced in The Flying Horse, but drinking in the Brummel just didn't have the same feel anymore. It was from that moment on that drinking came about chasing that buzz, wanting it to feel as good as those two weeks in Spain.

The next morning, things finally caught up with him. The hangover finally set in. Maybe it was the change in environment or the fact he was back to his old man beers over his swanky Bacardi's, but he was a state. It was, most likely, the worst hangover he had experienced thus far in his career, the kind that makes people say, "never again", as he himself would come to say a lot over the next 30+ years. But it seemed a small price to pay, as he had done it. The test was passed and he was an established drinker at the age of 18.

Driving, done.
Drinking, done.

Time to move on. What was Andrew "gonna" do next?

<u>Chapter 3</u>

Serendipity

Before writing each chapter of this book, I spend some time talking with my Dad in order to have a complete understanding of the story I intend to convey. It's been an incredibly eye-opening experience for me to be able to have such in-depth, serious discussions with a man who I've only ever known to be a clown. We sit down, I open the voice memo app on my phone, press record and we start discussing all the key points the next chapter should hit upon. I also make some shorthand notes on my laptop, interpreting what is being said in a structure that more easily lends itself to being translated into legible text. These pseudo-interviews usually last around half an hour which, for someone like Andrew, is ample time to fill me in on the details of all the necessary stories.

Quite often, Christine, my Mum, will also be present at these chats, sometimes coming in and out at various points of the conversation, to either back up a point or interject her own version of events. It seemed quite natural at this point of the story, then, to discuss the time in Andrew's life where he first met Christine, how they fell deeply in love with each other very quickly, and how alcohol would play its role in their relationship. It may, at times, seem quite an aside to have this love story feature so prominently in a story about a man's affair with addiction, but I feel it is absolutely necessary to have a thorough understanding of the couple's relationship and the roots of said relationship to understand how alcohol played its part in creating rifts between the two, essentially playing off each other to be the most important thing in Andrew's life.

So, for the following chapter, I asked for the story of the two meeting from Christine's perspective, allowing us to see the story without the beer-tinted glasses on and to understand how drink wasn't an element on the other side of the coin. Following that, I asked my Dad to tell the story from his point of view, to flesh out his feelings towards such a deep, true and meaningful relationship. Or, *relationships*, as it were.

. . . .

Friday, October 28th, 1983 - Christine Slinger was seated in the Craven Heifer, Kelbrook, with her mother, Doris, and her stepfather. Doris and her husband had encouraged the 17-year-old Christine to come along with them for the evening to the Heifer, making the trip from their home in Earby, because "there's a group of right good-looking lads that go in there on a Friday night." Being the last of her friends to snag herself a boyfriend, this was enough to convince her to go along and see these "lads" for herself. They stood at the bar for a while, the two adults sipping beers and wines, while Christine drank soft drinks, staying eagle eyed for these eligible bachelors, who she hoped would appear shortly.

Eventually, a group of young men entered the pub, got themselves a pint each from the bar and made their way to their usual spot, surrounding the jukebox, feeding coins into it, blasting out Iron Maiden, Def Leppard, Metallica, etc. Doris clocks them at first and points them out to Christine. She turns to look over her shoulder and sees our eponymous hero; "Oh my God, that's Andrew Dickin!" In a nervous panic, she quickly turned back round and pretended not to have noticed the boy she so fancied. She didn't know what else she could do. Going over and trying to strike up a conversation with him while he was surrounded by his friends was far too intimidating, so she quickly decided pretending to be invisible would be the best course of action. But it failed. Andrew had already caught her sneaky glance and decided to come over and speak to Christine and her family. The conversation was brief and awkward, with Christine not really knowing what to say and having the added pressure of her mother and stepfather being stood at the bar with her. After their fleeting chat, Andrew and his friends left and made their usual Friday-night trip to the Brummel, to commence the standard weekend binge. Andrew had another aim, too, which we will get to shortly.

As can be gleaned from the above, Christine was already well aware of Andrew before this night and had had an attraction to him for quite some time. They didn't mix in similar circles at school, but she knew who he was and had certainly developed a fancy for him. In her words, "he was gorgeous." But their first conversation probably didn't live up to the expectations that a young girl may fantasise about.

It was after school one day and Christine and her best friend Ingrid waited, as usual, for the last bus, as this was always the quiet one. The loud, impatient, popular kids would have got on the first bus home and neither girl enjoyed the company of those kids very much, so waiting a little longer to ride home in peace felt like a small price to pay. As they found their seat, side by side on the lower deck of the bus, Andrew spotted them and came and took the seat in front of them. He admits now that he actually fancied both of them - he must have seen it as a chance to break the ice with two possible love interests. But he didn't only break the ice, he shattered it into a thousand pieces with what would come next. He turned to face them with a huge grin on his face and dropped the following proverbial turd in the punch bowl: "Have you ever had a hot, sweaty fanny around your neck?" Stunned and shocked by this vulgarity, the pair replied, "absolutely not!"

"Yeah you have, when you were born." And with that, Andrew had introduced himself to the woman he would spend the rest of his life with. I mean, how could anybody resist such alluring charm and wit? Apparently, he had just learned the joke that day and couldn't wait to test it out on everybody he came across, perhaps not understanding that a couple of young girls wouldn't be as impressed as he himself had been. Despite opening in such a catastrophically bad manner, Christine, along with all her 14-year-old naivety, still fancied him, while it probably didn't wash quite as well with Ingrid, who simply replied, "well actually, I was a C-section" (Andrew tells me he didn't even know what that was at the time. Like I said, different circles). But Christine had fancied him right through school and a poor joke wasn't going to tarnish that.

Years later, Christine discovered, through friends of friends, that Andrew spent every Friday night (and every Saturday night, and every Sunday night…) at the Brummel and so, a week after their encounter at the Craven Heifer, four days before her 18th birthday, she made an excuse to tag along with a friend from college, Bev, who also frequented the Brummel on a Friday night. Just about everybody did. It was the "hip" place, the place to be on a weekend for the under 25 generation. They arrived early, giving Christine plenty of time to build up some "Dutch Courage", the kind of confidence delivered only through the medium of alcohol. She wasn't much of a drinker herself, and so it didn't take much for her to be on the tipsy side and feeling ready to pounce on her target. A couple of hours passed by before Andrew made his appearance, with the same group of friends he'd been with a week earlier at the Heifer. Being the creatures of habit that they were, they got their drinks and headed straight for the jukebox, where they'd planned to spend the rest of the evening.

As the night progressed, the pair made occasional eye contact, but neither had the nerve to make the first move. Andrew's confidence from the previous week, to go straight over and start up a conversation, was probably dampened by the presence of Christine's friends that he didn't know.

A table full of girls chatting away is a daunting thing for any young man, intoxicated or not. However, Christine was starting to see the night slipping through her fingers with every minute that passed without striking up a conversation. She felt as though she was blowing her perfect opportunity to snag him. This led to her making a very brash and uncharacteristic move. As Andrew made his way back from the bar, he passed by her table, at which point Christine made a snap decision to grab his backside. She was almost shocked at herself, that she would do such a bold thing, without giving it a second's thought. And at first, it seemed to have all been for nothing. He didn't even react. He carried on walking, pint in hand back to his spot at the jukebox. But little did she know, Andrew was just as shocked as she was. More so, in fact.

At this point, I would just like to back things up slightly and refocus on Andrew: What his feelings were towards Christine, his personal endeavours in finding love and, of course, his weekends at the Brummel.

Andrew was stood by the jukebox at The Craven Heifer with a group of friends. It was Friday night and as tradition dictated, they would drink a few pints here, being their local, before setting off for Earby, to get to The Brummel, where they would continue their drinking unabated. As they stood and discussed the kind of things that seem important at 18 (so and so got with so and so, have you heard the new Van Halen album?), he noticed a group of three people stood at the other end of the room. He quickly realised that he knew the older couple among the trio and made his way over to say hello. He had become friendly with Doris and her husband through their weekend patronage at the Heifer and had grown fond of them during that time. It was then that he noticed Christine Slinger was the third member of the party. He had been attracted to her throughout school (see 'sweaty fanny' story) and quickly came to the realisation that Doris was her mother. Feeling the awkward-ness emanating from Christine, clearly embarrassed by the fact her crush was closer to her Mum than he was to her, he left them to their evening and went back to his friends. They quickly drank up and moved on to the Brummel.

Andrew was particularly excited to be heading there this Friday. Not only because it was his favourite drinking establishment, but because he had got wind that a girl he had a thing for would be there that night. I suppose you may assume the beer would have the same Dutch courage effect it would have on Christine a week later, but who would tell the difference in Andrew? Intoxicated was his natural state on a Friday evening. And besides, as he was soon to find out, Al did not impart any knowledge about attracting women on him this evening. He was more focused on Andrew's continued training.

Securing their territory at the Brummel at the ol' jukebox, he saw the girl he was after. As a result of his early passions, Andrew could drink, everyone had been made aware of that, but pulling girls was a whole different ball game, and the two skill sets did not rub together for Andrew. He saw the girl he was hoping to impress. He said to his mates, "this is the night I'm going to pull her." So, he plucked up all the courage he could muster and made his way over to where she was standing, surrounded by her friends. She turned to acknowledge him. He froze completely. "hello, I, er…" With his forehead dampening, he continued, "what's erm… so…" She stared blankly back at him. What felt like hours passed by in seconds, until he turned and walked away, a complete and utter failure of an attempt at attracting the opposite sex. It seemed Andrew had put that much effort into building up his drinking repertoire, talking to girls had taken a back seat… right at the very back.

For the following week, Andrew felt scarred by the experience. Not only had he not managed to impress the girl he was trying to, but all her friends stood by and watched his public display of defeat, not to mention the grief he got from his own friends. Nonetheless, it wouldn't put him off his weekly ritual, he would still be at the Brummel on Friday, that's where Al would be, afterall.

Friday came around and off Andrew and his mates went. If you visit a place in such a ritualistic manner as to be there every week at the same time, you learn the names and the faces of all the regulars, so it came as a surprise to see the face of a girl he had never seen in there before. A face he knew, but not one of the Brummel crowd. It was Christine Slinger. For the next while, he would cast cursory glances at her from across the pub, trying to build up the courage to say something, but his defeat from the week before had left him with ice cold feet and so cursory glances would have to do for now. The night proceeded, Andrew drinking his usual fill and pumping coins into the jukebox. He was making his way back from the bar when he suddenly felt somebody grab him by the backside. He quickly realised it was Christine, and he couldn't believe what just happened. Not wanting to make a fool of himself, he carried on as though nothing had happened. In his mind, he was stunned by it. He arrived back at his perch and told his mates what had just happened. Naturally, they didn't believe him. Christine Slinger wouldn't do something like that! She was quiet and smart and far too good for him! But she had done it, and Andrew knew it and he knew that he had to act upon it, rather than just pretending nothing had happened. He took one last gulp for good luck and made his way over to where she was standing. He was starting to feel nauseous from the cocktail of nerves and beer swilling around his stomach. Sweaty palms in check, he asked her if she wanted to go outside to talk. So far so good, he had at least managed to speak legible sentences to her. She agreed and they made their way outside where the conversation between them started to flow. Amazed by how well he was doing, the toxic combination in his stomach became too much. "Excuse me a minute" he said to her as he vaulted over the wall just in time to hurl up his stomach contents. As Gordie Lachance would say in Stand by Me, "Total barf-o-rama."

Despite this mishap, the pair got what they both wanted. They connected instantly and spent the rest of the evening together, with Andrew walking her home at the end of the night. Christine was wearing a pair of very high shoes, which were hurting her feet more than she let on, but she decided she could endure the pain. It was worth it to be walking and talking with him. Andrew, on the other hand, was having a revelation of his own; during this walk, he realised he wanted to spend the rest of his life with

Christine. It seems cheesy and overly romantic to state such a thing, but he recalls that he had that exact feeling at that time and was shocked to realise that, at the age of 18, he had found his "one."

The following evening, Christine was going to 'The Cats Whiskers' to celebrate her 18th birthday (the coming Monday) and she invited Andrew to come along, which, of course, he accepted. It must have been strange for Christine's friends and family who went that night, as they barely had sight of her since her and Andrew spent the entire evening together upstairs at the Whiskers. After that, they saw each other every day without fail.

Naturally, this seemed to drive a wedge between Andrew and Al, who grew very jealous about the ever-growing relationship between the two. Of course, Andrew would spend *some* time with him, having a few drinks wherever the courting couple went - he wasn't ready to abandon his training that early - but seeing each other every day meant interrupting Andrew's weekly rituals. It seemed he had actually found what he was gonna do next and it wasn't drinking. But Al soon managed to worm his way back in and made Andrew start to realise what he was missing. He eventually persuaded him to start to visit the pub after spending time with Christine. They would spend the evening together, perhaps going for a meal, which Andrew would generously pay for. He would only drink half a pint of lager at the meal and then he would drive home. They would then go back to Christine's house where the family cat would maul him for a while and then, upon leaving, he would make it back in time to get a couple of pints down his neck before last orders. Christine had no idea he was doing this and wasn't really aware that Andrew had such a relationship with booze.

Having come together in November and quickly realising their love for each other, by March the following year, the pair were engaged. Five years would go by from then before they got married, during which time they didn't live together, still living with their parents and saving money to eventually get a home of their own (which they did a year before tying the knot. They still didn't live together then and would instead spend the next year working on the house, getting it ready for when they were married). Any social event that the pair attended together would be an excuse for Andrew to drink, which he did with growing intensity. That feeling of not wanting the party to end that Andrew felt after returning from his first lads' holiday would arise constantly. He would always be the last to leave, wanting everybody to stay out and keep going with him. But to Christine and everybody else, it hardly appeared to be a problem. In their words, everybody their age drank. It was just the social norm and I suppose it remains that way to this day and so at a young age, the realisation that a problem may be bubbling away under the surface just didn't come. There was, however, one incident before they were married, in which Christine planted the seeds of belief that Andrew had a drink problem. Neither can recall the situation picture perfectly, but my Dad tells it like this:

Talking to Christine - "We were at your house one night and it was quite late, and we were sitting on the sofa and you said to me "you have a problem with drink, don't you?" I said "I don't have a problem, that's who I am. I enjoy drinking and I am definitely not going to stop, so if you don't like it or you've got a problem with it, then you better get used to it, because I'm not changing for anybody."

As will be revealed throughout the remainder of this story, and indeed, this chapter, Christine was of course correct. Andrew did have a problem. And these were just the early days. The issue was just a sapling at this stage. It would bloom over the coming months and years and Christine would try her very best to maintain it. She loved him and didn't want to lose him.

Andrew's stag do was quite a standard affair. He didn't do anything extravagant, his friends didn't plan a coach trip anywhere, he simply wanted to go to his favourite places: The Heifer and The Brummel. So that's what they did. Anybody who wanted to tag along could do. It goes without saying, Andrew got incredibly drunk, having to be carried home and placed on to his sofa by his mates. But it was his stag do, so I suppose it was to be expected. What wasn't to be expected though was his attitude on the big day. Their wedding was incredibly picturesque, taking place in Kelbrook's beautiful church and being attended by a very large audience of friends and family. They were then treated to a helicopter ride over to the Stirk House Hotel for the reception, which was also where they would be spending their first night as husband and wife. It really was a perfect day for them. That was, until Andrew's insatiable craving set in. All his friends went straight to the bar to begin the day's drinking, but Andrew couldn't as he had to stay outside while the photographer took their wedding photos. His jealousy at the fact the guests were populating the bar continued to grow as the photographer took more and more photos, moving them to different positions and retaking shots. He became incredibly agitated, knowing that his friends were possibly on their 2nd, or maybe even their 3rd drinks by this point and he was still as sober as a judge. Christine could sense a change in him and was very shocked to see that a thirst for booze could bring out this side of him she rarely saw. Again, his problem with drink was presenting itself to her, on this, the happiest day of their lives.

Quick aside - It really was the happiest day of their lives and they couldn't be more thrilled to have committed themselves to each other for the rest of their lives, but it was becoming increasingly clear to Christine that Andrew had another love in his life.

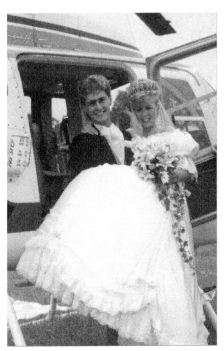

Once the photos were taken and the couple had spent time doing the rounds, shaking hands, hugging people and thanking them for attending, Andrew was finally able to join his friends in a serious bout of drinking, playing catch up with them by drinking as much as humanly possible in a short period of time. Christine would barely see him for the rest of the day, as she continued to move around the room, spending time with guests and dancing.

Towards the end of the night, guests were starting to leave in the order they generally do: the tired grandparents had already left, the work colleagues shortly after them, the distant family would then follow suit until the core of the party was made up of close friends and family, enjoying the remaining moments of what had been a very beautiful wedding day. But as the numbers thinned even more, it grew ever more clear that, in typical Andrew fashion, he was not ready for the party to be over. The bar was still open, so why not carry on? But even Andrew's friends, who were not too sober themselves, encouraged him to call it a night. "It's your wedding night, Andrew. You have your wife waiting for you to go to the room you have here and do what newlyweds do!" But the bar is open! Don't you understand! We *must* carry on the party! His defiance was strong. It was clear he only wanted one thing, and it wasn't to go to his wedding bed.

Eventually, they managed to pry him away, his inhibitions weakened greatly by the level of consumption and he stumbled his way to their hotel room where, Christine claims, he was so intoxicated that he could barely remove her dress. Again, the day was wonderful in many regards. They both looked amazing in their wedding attire, the venue was perfect, so many people had come to witness it, everybody had enjoyed themselves (some more than others), but it will always remain a question of how things could have played out different had Andrew been able to keep Al at arm's length, instead of embracing him in such a fervent manner when he should have been doing so with his wife.

If the seeds of Christine's worry had been planted on the evening of that frank conversation and the tree began to take root on their wedding day, it would be in full growth by the end of their honeymoon in Cyprus, where she finally got to see Andrew revert back to those days in Spain with Nibs and Nanny and the rest. It took only a matter of hours for him to be stuck into the booze, fully entering party mode at the hotel bar, while she was in the room, unpacking. She simply decided to leave him to it. He was already too far gone by the time she could join him and trying to have any form of normal conversation with him was completely out of the question. So she stayed in the room, continued to unpack and then called it a night. Andrew made his way back to the room in the early hours of the following morning, barely coherent and excitedly telling Christine that the bartender was a supporter of some football team or another and telling her about all the people he had met while under the influence. He babbled, "this is going to be a brilliant holiday." But Christine just wanted to go back to sleep and start afresh the day after.

As it turns out, Andrew was right, they did have an excellent holiday. Neither had ever experienced a climate as hot as Cyprus, spending most of the daylight hours at the beach, thoroughly enjoying being in the company of their freshly married partners. But as soon as the beer and wine were poured, the other side of Andrew emerged, as though he was behaving differently to try and impress Al and keep him happy, Christine growing ever more aware of the issues that she would face if she couldn't put a lid on this situation and fast. But as Andrew had told her in the past, "I'm not changing for anybody." It is a very good thing that Christine was not a big drinker herself, and that she realised it was possible for Andrew to change. Had this not been the case, the story of recovery that is yet to unfold would likely never have taken place.

Chapter 4

Back to the Future

I am a huge fan of artist/director David Lynch. A man whose films and works focus on very surreal qualities and deep, rich meanings. He is somewhat of an inspiration in a lot of facets of my life, most recently, through his devotion and belief in transcendental meditation. This spiritual dedication of his can often be glimpsed through his work, or at least interpreted through some messages forecast within. Arguably, David's most famous work would be the hit 90's soap/mystery/whodunnit show, Twin Peaks. A show of incredibly dense layers of mystery, intrigue, branching stories, complex, other-worldly qualities, and an incredible cast of oddball characters, each as rich and endearing as the last. This off-the-wall show made David Lynch into a household name in the 90's, a rare feat for a surrealist artist who employs dark and mysterious qualities so heavily.

Twin Peaks started with one event: The murder of Laura Palmer. It is said within the show, "Laura is the one." The one in which everything else sprouts out. All the qualities I previously mentioned about the show grew out of this one event and in real-world terms, catapulted Lynch and his work to new levels he would never have imagined, all thanks to the idea he had of Laura Palmer, and her death.

The reason I am telling you this is because the ensuing chapter of Andrew's story grew out of one event (that, and because I will take any opportunity to talk about Lynch and Twin Peaks). An event which, at the time, seemed to be a cataclysmic disaster for my Dad, Mum, myself, born in 1993 and Chris, born in 1991. But, as you will see throughout this story, from that one event came opportunities that may never have presented themselves had this event not occurred. They changed our lives in ways we could never have expected. But to get there, my Dad would have to experience incredible lows. It is a true story that presents the fact that, out of bad, can come good. Incredible, unexpected goodness that can quite literally change a person's life. If things in your life seem bad and it feels like you can't get much lower, it is always possible to bring yourself not only back to the surface, but to go way beyond that, to heights that seemed impossible from down in the gutter.

. . . .

March 1994 - Andrew and Christine had been married for 5 years now and had been living in the house they bought together and spent a year renovating in Barnoldswick. They had their first child, Christopher in June 1991, before I came along in April 1993. We lived a comfortable life in this house, Mum and Dad learning as they went along what having two young boys would be like to try and balance, but doing an incredible job. We certainly weren't a wealthy family, but we had enough to live happy lives and to be a close, growing family. Andrew was still working as a self-employed decorator at the time, doing work alongside his Dad, George. Credited most likely to hereditary issues, Andrew would suffer occasionally with a bad back, much like his Dad and his sister, who experience similar problems, but his day-to-day working life certainly didn't aid in this matter. Little did he know, the pain was an indication of the ticking time bomb within his spine.

One night, Christine was out visiting her Grandma Katie, my great-grandmother. Andrew was sitting in the living room, having a couple of beers and watching football on the TV. As a 1-year old baby will often do, I started crying loudly, upstairs in my cot. Andrew put his beer down and came upstairs to try and get me to calm down and go back to sleep. He came into the room and reached down to pick me up. He cradled me for a while and made some of those stupid baby talk sounds that every adult thinks is exactly what a baby wants to hear. It must have worked, because I ceased making the awful racket I was making, and Andrew went to put me back in my cot. Just as he was laying me down, he was struck. He describes it as feeling like he had been shot in the back. The timer had finished its countdown and had detonated. Andrew collapsed to the floor, beside my cot, paralysed by indescribable pain. I remained in my cot, a silent witness, as Andrew lay on the floor unable to process the physical reality of what was happening, and the mental realisation that his back had done exactly as it had warned. All of a sudden, he had gone from having a normal evening at home to being in so much pain that he couldn't bear to move a muscle. But with nobody in the house who could do anything to assist him, and with no idea how much longer Christine would be out for, he had to take matters into his own hands. He forced himself through the pain of turning over onto his hands and knees, a movement that elevated the pain to a higher level. In absolute agony and fear, he started to slowly crawl out of my room, aiming to get to the telephone downstairs. He slowly made his way down, one step at a time, dripping with sweat. Eventually, through agonising effort, he made it to the phone and called Christine at her grandma's house (of course, there were no mobile phones then). "You're going to have to come home. I don't know what's happened, but I can't walk, I need you."

Andrew initially thought that this would put him out of work for a couple of weeks at most, which would have been devastating for a family with only one source of income - with Christine being a full-time mother of myself and Chris. But these initial concerns paled in comparison to the eventual reality of being out of work for eight months. A very long time indeed to have absolutely no money coming into the household. Christine would make a pot of stew at the beginning of the week and that would have to suffice for the next seven days. Grandparents would buy essential supplies for us such as nappies, milk and other crucial items needed for the care of a 1 and a 3-year old. On top of all this, Christine had the fresh burden of being Andrew's carer, as he couldn't move from his makeshift bed in the living room, which consisted of the sofa cushions on the floor. He had no choice but to live in the living room, unable to make his way upstairs and hardly even able to maneuver around the ground floor of the house. He even had to do his business in my potty, which I very kindly loaned to him. I'm good like that. The doctor came to see him, Dr Evans, who entered the house to find

Andrew laying almost in the fetal position, with his back against the sofa. He had found a position there that seemed to relieve some level of pain, but he couldn't move from it. Dr Evans, clearly seeing the torture that the man was facing, sat on the sofa beside him and began to stroke his head, like you would a wounded animal in a display of sympathy. He was prescribed the strongest painkillers available. So strong, in fact, that after a while, Dr Miller, the head of the surgery, a man Andrew had never even heard of, called and asked him to stop taking the painkillers, as they were far too addictive and could lead to serious medical complications.

Of course, whilst on such strong medication, alcohol cannot be consumed and so the painkillers acted as a wedge between him and Al, who he saw very little of over this 8-month period, only having the occasional treat once he was off the meds. But he would see people walking by the window, on their way down to The Strategy, the pub just down the road from the house. At first, he felt intense jealousy towards the fact those people were on their way to enjoy a few drinks with their friends, but that jealousy soon took on another form; a jealousy of the simple fact they could walk *anywhere*, not just to the pub. And so, for the first time since being 18, Andrew wasn't a drinker. The first silver lining to emerge from this incredibly dense clouding that had formed over his life. Instead, he would have to continue to lay on the floor of the living room, watching Chris Evans' Big Breakfast of a morning and comedy VHS's of an evening.

Life continued in this way for the months following March, with constant doctor's visits, scans and different courses of medication in an attempt to get him back on his feet. We were quickly running out money and Christine was run ragged having to care for the three of us. One day in the summer, Andrew received a telephone call from a man called Kevin Pickles. Andrew had befriended Kevin through spending time as a trucker's mate, essentially going on long distance journeys with wagon drivers to keep them company and assist where they can on certain jobs. He had been with Kev a number of times after school, helping him wherever he could, and the pair really got on well. Kev had heard about the condition Andrew was in and called with a proposition. "Now then Andrew, I hear you're not so good."

"No, Kev. I'm in a very bad way. I can't even walk!"

"Nay, that's no good. Well, I've got an idea if you fancy it, get you out t'house. I've a job to do over Manchester way tomorrow, Cheetham Hill. Fancy coming along for't ride, just see how you go on?" It seemed like a bad idea at first, but he decided to go along with him to see how it went, as Kev said. They went the next day to Manchester, with Andrew experiencing a lot of pain, sitting in the wagon cab, but also thinking how great it was to simply be out of the house and chatting to someone else. After making the delivery and driving home, Kev told him that if he fancied it, he had a couple more jobs coming up and he would gladly have him along for the ride. And so over the next few weeks and months, Andrew made a number of these trips, still in excruciating pain but wanting to get out more and more now that Kev had got him moving. They would call at service stations along the way for a rest and Kev would have to park his huge, articulated lorry right at the pedestrian entrance to the services, simply so Andrew would have less distance to travel to get to the restroom.

One of the last trips Andrew made with Kev required an overnight stay in the lorry. They had done a few jobs of this nature over the period but, on this particular occasion, they stayed at the end of a long country lane, where, at the other end, stood a pub. Kev suggested that they attempt to walk up the lane to enjoy a couple of pints. Andrew was off his painkillers by this point, so an evening with Al was certainly possible, but of course, he had a huge obstacle in his way. Spurred on both by the thought of accomplishing something as huge as the walk and the thought of the amber reward at the other end, he agreed and they slowly set off up the lane, a journey that was far longer than any Andrew had made on foot in months. As they neared the pub doors and the smell of ale started to waft over his nostrils, he had a sudden realisation that he had nearly finished the walk. He couldn't believe it. It felt like a miracle to him. After spending months struggling to stand, having to use a potty for his business and not being able to work a single day, here he was having walked the full length of a country lane and about to enjoy the bounteous reward of a few pints. This was truly a milestone in his recovery, and it was all thanks to Kev.

Andrew and Kev continued to make these journeys for a good while, before Andrew decided he wanted to stretch his legs elsewhere, now that he could maneuver somewhat. He thanked Kev for reaching out to him and for essentially getting him going again and called it a day on his short-lived trucker's mate revival. He decided, instead, to explore the world of car sales. Ever since he was a young boy, cars had fascinated him, evidenced by his aching desire to drive all those years ago and since reaching adulthood, he had fancied himself as being a car salesman, but had blotted out the idea, considering it impossible. He wasn't very well educated, he couldn't read, he couldn't write, qualities he had decided were essential to be able to achieve this dream. So it remained exactly that, a dream, one that he'd ponder endlessly when he was well enough to put his overalls back on and get back to decorating. But for now, at least, he could go and be a fly-on-the-wall at his cousin's garage.

David O'Neill owned a forecourt in Andrew's hometown of Kelbrook where he sold second-hand cars. His brother, Shaun, also worked there. Having lived so close to each other as children, Andrew had a very close relationship with his cousins and admired them for their work, wanting to do the same for himself. He decided to contact them to see if they would mind him coming down to the garage and just observing how the business works, and maybe helping out here and there wherever he could. Of course, they had no issue with that and were looking forward to seeing Andrew, since he had been seen so rarely since his tremendous set back. Christine dropped him off at the garage the next day and he spent the next few weeks learning the ropes, seeing how the job operated and being fascinated to see behind the curtain of a career he so longed for.

Andrew arrived one morning, made a coffee and went to sit in David's office, to see what was happening that day. They discussed the sales that would be finalised that day, the cars that would be coming in soon and other daily operations of the garage. Then, David happened to mention that Preston's BMW Dealership in Colne, a 15-minute drive from Barnoldswick, was looking for an overnight security guard. "You see, the first of the month is when the new car shipments come into the showroom, so they're short of someone to do the night shift, just basically keeping an eye out", David explained.

"Well, I'll do it, I've nowt on" Andrew replied, excitedly. He saw Preston's as the holy grail of car dealerships for the area. A sophisticated car brand such as BMW, with high class clients, in a very pristine showroom. It was the pinnacle of his salesman dreams.

"How can you do it, with the state you're in? You're lucky to be able to get out of the house as it is," David said, not forgetting that despite his get-up-and-go attitude, Andrew was still not deemed in a state to be working anywhere.

"Yeah but, I'll be reyt, nothing's going to happen with me there. It's not like I'm going to have to chase folk or owt."

"But Andrew, in an ideal world, they need someone who can start tonight and do it for the next week."

"That's fine, I'll ask David Entwistle if I can borrow one of his Special uniforms and get over there!" David Entwistle was Andrew's sister,

Kath's husband, at the time and worked as a Special for the police, who have smart, official looking uniforms, which Andrew thought would be perfect for the job.

"Right well, I'll ring them, if you're sure?" David called them there and then. "Okay, get yourself over there for 7pm. They'll have ya." It might not be the salesman position he was thinking of, but it was a foot in the door at least!

Keen to impress and to learn his duties, Andrew arrived at the showroom early. To his delight, he didn't have to stand for the evening and simply had to sit in a chair from 7pm to 7am, keeping an eye out for anybody pulling onto the forecourt or any suspicious behaviour. He was even offered the company of Simon Preston's dog, Roger. Simon was the co-owner of the business and his dog was a big, strong, Staffordshire bull terrier, the kind that gets a bad name for being violent, but actually craves human attention and affection more than anything else. Still, if you saw Roger running at you in the middle of the night while trying to pry open the locked doors of a car dealership, you'd drop your back in one half-less than no time.

7pm came around and so started Andrew's first shift as a Nocturnal Security Officer. Through the window, he could see the Colne town hall clock, which he kept one eye on as the un-eventful evening crept by. He quickly discovered that, to his nature, Roger wanted his attention and so he jumped all over him frequently throughout the night. Funny as it seemed and although he enjoyed playing with him, it hurt his back a great deal every time he pounced on him and so it wasn't really an ideal situation. However, he didn't complain and continued the job unabated. One night, around midnight, a car pulled onto the forecourt, the first such action Andrew had seen in his position. He moved as quickly as his back would allow him to get into a "hiding" position behind a car in the showroom, with enough of a view to see the man stepping out of the vehicle. It turned out to be a well-known businessman from the area, who had ordered a number of cars for himself and his family and was simply coming to look in at his new purchases through the showroom window. Andrew's realisation of who the gentleman was came just as Roger decided he wanted to play with Andrew. He leapt onto him, pushing Andrew to the floor, where, of course, he couldn't get up, due to his back pain (and the fact a heavy staffy was now climbing all over him). He wrestled with the dog, who of course thought he was joining in his game, eventually getting him to back off, whereafter he slowly got himself back to his feet. He looked out and saw the car had left the forecourt and the man was nowhere to be seen. Years later, Andrew happened to bump into the son of said businessman in a pub (of course), who somehow got around to the subject of Preston's BMW dealership. He said "my Dad came home from there one night. He'd been to look at the cars we'd ordered, and he said that he saw a security officer wrestling with a dog inside the showroom, if you can believe it!" Of course, he believed it. He confessed to being the phantom dog wrestler, much to the amusement of the whole room.

The week went by, Andrew enjoying his time as an NSO. He arrived at the showroom one evening, early as ever and was getting ready for his shift when Simon Preston approached him and asked, "what's your plan with your back, Andrew?" to which he told him he wasn't sure. He had a make-or-break operation coming up, which he was terrified of. He didn't know how successful it would be, if it would fix the issue permanently and whether he would ever be able to return to work as a decorator, which seemed incomprehensible in his current state. He could not see a clear road ahead that would lead him back to that position. For now, he felt blessed to be doing what he was. There wasn't much opportunity to work in his condition, so to be doing so was very important to him and to us all as a family, also.

A few weeks passed following his time watching cars and wrestling dogs and Andrew had gone once again to see David and Shaun in Kelbrook. He was still calling in a couple of times a week, soaking up more and more of the world of car sales. He sat in David's office for the usual catch up, but David looked at him and smiled. "Andrew, I've got something to tell you," he said, smile widening.

"What's that?" Andrew replied, with no idea what could possibly come next.

"Simon and Richard have told me they're going to offer you a new position at Preston's. They want you to be a trainee salesman." Andrew couldn't believe what he was hearing. The last eight months flashed before him: Out of work, no money to provide for his family, agonising pain, month after month of misery and he felt like at that very moment, somebody had handed him a winning lottery ticket. He'd taken the job as security man under the impression that that was as high up the Preston's ladder he would ever climb. He had no inclination that he would be offered his dream job, because of it. Him, an illiterate, out of work, self-employed decorator.

He was asked to go over to visit the showroom shortly after that for an informal chat/interview to finalise the proposal. He just walked in the door when Simon saw him from his office and shouted, "ey up, Andy's here! You'll be doing these soon!" holding up an intimidating looking piece of paper.

"What's that?" Andrew asked.

"Order forms." He had a sudden realisation that this job would take a lot of hard work. He would have to try his best to appear professional, doing work that involved reading and writing. This was something unlike he had ever done before. Simon called him into his office, where he officially offered him the job. "Go and have your operation, get yourself sorted, and when you're ready, you're going to come here and we're going to make a salesman of you. Just get yourself sorted and we'll be waiting." He could not believe that this man who he admired so greatly was offering him such a kindness. He was so overwhelmed by the situation that he cried on his way back home. The tears were a product of incredible heartfelt gratitude. He was about to step into the greatest job he would ever have. He would be able to provide for his family, once again. His parents and Christine's parents could cease having to buy them essentials, life would not only return to normal, but it had the potential to be better than it had ever been before. As all these joyous thoughts rushed through his head on the car journey home, his back twinged, and he suddenly remembered, "I've got to get this thing sorted first."

The day of the operation came and Andrew was sat in his ward at the hospital. There were three other men in the room, all waiting for operations of their own. The gentleman across from Andrew called out to him, "what are you in for then, lad?"

"I'm here for an operation on my back" Andrew shakily replied, nerves for the coming operation absolutely wracking him.

"Ah yeah, I've had one of them" the man replied, "that's why I'm back again."

"Same here", the man next to Andrew said.

"Yeah, and me, too," the third man said. Just in case he wasn't nervous enough already, the thought that the operation wouldn't even solve the issue was now playing on his mind and worsening his nerves tenfold. After a while of quiet contemplation for what was about to happen, Dr. Beard, Andrew's doctor, entered the room. "Right, young man, let's get you down there" he said, directing Andrew to get himself ready and to make his way to the operation theatre. "Now, before we do this, are you sure you want to go through with it? This is keyhole surgery and as you've been made aware of on the waver, there are a number of high risks involved. It's up to you, we can either do this now, or I can give you an epidural."

"That one", Andrew replied, not unlike a Matt Lucas sketch show character.

"The epidural?"

"Yes, that one. I didn't even know that was an option!" So instead of the operation, Andrew had the epidural, a method of delivering an anesthetic to stop pain signals traveling from the spine to the brain. As soon as he was cleared to leave and he arrived home, he called Simon Preston and said, "I'm home, I didn't have the op, but I'm ready."

Later that same day, Richard Preston, Simon's cousin and business partner called and invited Andrew to attend a BMW closed auction the following day. This is essentially where the officially licensed BMW dealerships bid on used BMW stock, a very important, key aspect of any car dealership. Andrew agreed to go along with him, excited that his first day on the job would be spent with one of the business owners, attending to something very important and learning directly from him. What he didn't know until he arrived at the auction was that Richard had intended on giving him the paddle and letting Andrew do the bidding, deciding which stock Preston's should purchase and how much they should spend on it. Such responsibility was handed to him on the first day, and he was absolutely thrilled.

After the excitement of the auction, Andrew started his trainee salesman job in earnest the day after. In his freshly pressed suit, he arrived early and was shown to his desk and taught the ropes. Although it was overwhelming, he felt like he was living in a dream. Things were moving so fast after eight seemingly endless months. He pushed all his nerves to one side and applied everything he could to his work, which led to his first sale within two days, an incredibly impressive feat for a man with no prior experience. He had hit the ground running, and Richard and Simon couldn't be happier. They later told him that people had doubted their choice in taking Andrew on on such a whim. But to be able to prove those naysayers wrong within 48 hours was a huge victory for them all.

Life for the Dickin family quickly began to change. We had enough expendable cash to get Christine her own car, meaning the couple would no longer have to share. Not only that, but Christine ended up with a receptionist job at Preston's, working two days a week, bringing in extra money and still allowing enough time in the week for her to do all the necessary "Mum" jobs. Andrew quickly established himself as a key member of the team, which was no easy task in such a competitive work environment, all salesmen trying to be at the top of the monthly sales chart.

Al was never far from thought, now that Andrew could drink again. Tuesday was Andrew's weekly day off and so Monday nights quickly became a bonus party night for Andrew, on top of the usual weekend binges. He would spend every Monday night with his good friend Alan Sagar, the proprietor of a local off-licence. With Andrew's newfound confidence and business-acclimated mind, they would drunkenly discuss between themselves how only "big-hitters" drink like they do. Only people with things to say and were interesting people, in other words. I'm not entirely sure of the logic behind this thought process, but I suppose that's the kind of thing that an intoxicated mind can convince itself of. So, they would drink to excess every Monday, meaning every Tuesday off that Andrew had was mostly wasted, in his incredibly hungover state, whiling away the day on the sofa. And it wasn't only with Alan on a Monday night that he would enter party mode: Sales targets met, Christmas parties, drinks after work on a Friday, company BBQ's, whatever the occasion, Andrew saw it as a golden opportunity to strengthen his relationship with Al.

With the training wheels off, the need to make a good impression subsided and with Andrew fully embedded into this new environment, he began to soar. He attended endless BMW corporate events, using his characteristic charm and wit to befriend some of the company's elite players, who were so impressed to find that Andrew worked for a dealership in a town like Colne, which is very small in comparison to the big city dealerships, where they would expect to find somebody of his calibre. He constantly had a great sales record, had return customers who wanted to deal with him exclusively and the rest of the team found that he was born into the role. But after a while, the apple cart started to wobble, and cracks started to appear in the foundations of Andrew's performance. Around a year into his work, things started to get on top of him. A combination of never saying no to a request and his impatience when it came to written work resulted in backlogged paperwork piling up. His overeager nature working against hum, the future started to look uncertain and Andrew was aware of that in himself. This rocked his confidence and his entire work performance suffered.

It was time to acknowledge the issue head-on, which fell on the shoulders of Richard. Andrew was busily working away at his desk, trying and failing to get on top of the mounting tasks. He pulled the seat out across from Andrew and sat down. "I don't think things are quite working properly, are they Andrew?" His heart sank. He knew things weren't great and he began to think to himself, "I knew this would happen eventually, but I was hoping it wouldn't be so soon." He started to feel his dream slipping away from him and he was on the verge of tears, right there, in the showroom, in front of one of the bosses. He bit his lip, and once Richard had left his desk, he continued to work, ashamed of himself and worrying about slipping back to the gutter.

Towards the end of the day, it was Simon's turn to talk to Andrew. Andrew still believes to this day that Simon is one of the greatest managers of a team he has ever experienced. He knows exactly how to maintain the balance of work and friendship and how to get the best out of each individual, which was perhaps what led to his next gesture. He sat down at Andrew's desk and said, "I'm sorry about this Andrew, but we really need to get things back on track for the company. I do have one suggestion, though. Have you ever heard of a man called Brian Tracy? He's an author." Asking Andrew if he's heard of an author is like asking a worm if he's heard of Mozart.

"No, I don't think so", Andrew replied, despondently, not really seeing where Simon was going and too busy feeling downtrodden.

"Well, he's written a book called 'The Psychology of Selling', which I happen to have on cassette. There are six tapes altogether and I really think you should listen to it. It might just turn things around for you." He said, as he placed the boxset on Andrew's desk.

"Thanks, I'll give them a go" Andrew replied, knowing full well he had no intentions of listening to some "self-help rubbish" - so naive. And so, on his way home, into the glovebox it went, to be forgotten about.

Nothing was set in stone yet and so Andrew still had his job for the time being. I suppose it was a warning in order to soften the blow when and if they had to pull the trigger. So, Andrew would still turn up to work every day in what felt like a fruitless endeavour. In a way, he'd already given up, following the news he'd been given. He had lost his confidence, and he could see no way of getting it back. Each morning he would arrive and Simon would say, "have you listened to those tapes yet, Andrew?"

"Oh no, I completely forgot, Simon!" Then the next day;

"Have you listened to those tapes yet, Andrew?"

"I had a lot on last night, so I didn't get around to it!" And the day after that;

"Have you listened to those tapes yet, Andrew?" and so on and so on, until eventually, Andrew came to the realisation that this endless cycle wouldn't cease until he listened to the god forsaken tapes. The weekend came around, as it does every week, and Andrew and Christine decided to have a Chinese take away, perhaps in an effort to try and boost Andrew's spirits. Afterall, there's nothing like a good dollop of MSG to chase the blues away. On his drive to Earby to pick up the food, Andrew finally caved, thinking, "Simon is definitely going to ask me on Monday if I've listened to those bloody tapes," so in went tape number one. The drive to Earby from Barnoldswick takes no more than five minutes, but this was enough time for Andrew to have his mind blown. So much so that, when he parked up outside the Jade Palace Chinese restaurant, he stayed seated in his car for the next 5 or 10 minutes, completely engrossed in Mr Tracy's inspiring words. This was the first time Andrew had ever experienced any form of self-help and he couldn't believe what he was hearing. It was like being handed the cheat book to sales. Do this, say that, write this, think that and bada-bing, sale accomplished. Following that evening, every car journey he made would include those six cassettes on a constant rotation, until all the cheat codes to success were ingrained in his mind. And the results were plain to see. He got through all his paperwork, he climbed back up the sales board, he continued to attend training seminars, impressing BMW bigwigs. His confidence was back in full stride and it saved him.

He wasn't let go from the company and managed to fully regain his position as a strong and essential member of the team, all thanks to a self-help book written by Brian Tracy, gifted to him by Simon.

Andrew stayed at Preston's for three years. He continued to grow his sales portfolio and really honed his skills as a professional car salesman. Due to a change in circumstances within the Preston's group, Andrew resigned. Although this was the best job he'd ever had, he felt this was the right move to make for himself and did it with full confidence, but that didn't stop him from being emotional over the decision. His journey home on his last day mirrored that of the day he first got the job four years prior; he cried. Preston's had been a life jacket when he needed it the most. It helped shape the rest of his life.

He spent the next few months and years continuing on as a car salesman. With the credentials under his belt to earn such a position, he no longer relied on sheer luck and circumstance and he went through a number of different establishments, working at some of the finest car dealerships in the area and beyond. But nothing compared to his first sales job, with his motivational gurus above him and the friends and people he had grown to care about surrounding him and so none of these jobs lasted.

Eventually, Andrew decided to call it a day. He had achieved and lived his dream. Everything else paled in comparison, so there was only one thing left for him to do and that was to pick up his paintbrush and go back to his trade.

Looking back to March 1994, when Andrew experienced the worst set back of his life to that point and it seemed his new, young family faced a dark future, little did he know that that one event, shrouded in pain, sadness and dread would lead him through four completely life changing years. And in a way, this time would come to serve as some form of metaphor for Andrew's life. As drink continued to dominate a large portion of his existence, things grew incredibly bleak. But, as the first chapter of this book has already told you, he came out of the other end of that bleakness. And as you will discover later, not only did he emerge from it, he soared way above it, achieving what he deemed impossible.

Chapter 5

The Law of Attraction

I remember when I first realised that my Mum was trying to get control over my Dad's drinking. When I was 17, I started working in a pub in Barnoldswick. I only did a couple of nights a week, starting out glass collecting until I was old enough to start pulling pints. I'd get home around midnight, or sometimes later, depending what had taken place at work that evening. When working at the weekend, more often than not, I would arrive home to find my Dad comatose on the floor, or on the sofa. The TV would be off, everywhere would be locked up and my Mum would already be in bed, but she would leave the wine bottle out next to him, I guess as a way to remind him how he ended up in that state when he eventually awoke and stumbled his way to bed. On the occasions he wasn't there upon returning home, I discovered that my Mum had been using a calendar, hung on the inside of a cupboard door in the kitchen to keep track of the days he had a drink. It was like one of those "X amount of days since the last accident" signs you often see in on screen depictions of factories or dangerous work environments. She never told me that's what she was doing, and I can't quite remember how I discovered it, but I quickly got into the tradition of checking the calendar whenever I got home late, feeling pleased and proud if it indicated no drink, or sad and disappointed if the opposite. Occasionally, there'd be a string of days where he hadn't had a drink, and I felt genuine elation and actual pride – a strange thing to feel towards a father, who should be saying those things of myself – but these were few and far between. More often than not, the calendar would be covered in crossed out blotches that denoted another night with Al. I was sad for my Dad, because it just meant that he'd had another evening ensnared in the booze trap, but I was much more sad for my Mum. It meant that she'd had another night spent watching my Dad party on his own, steadily slurring his speech before eventually crashing out onto the floor. Knowing that she was keeping track of the days like this highlighted to me that it was a growing problem for her and I became much more aware of the struggle she was silently facing, watching the man she loves slowly evaporating into a wine-scented world.

Of course, it's very difficult for me to put into words the actual emotions my mother experienced during these times. Such a personal and heartfelt battle can only be expressed by the person who lived it, not an onlooker, despite the fact I shared the same house as them. For that reason, I asked my Mum to put into her own words her thoughts on Andrew's drinking career. She was incredibly nervous and apprehensive, both because she has never attempted to write in this fashion before, worried that people wouldn't find her words interesting and also because she was admitting truths that she kept locked away for so long. But once she'd finished writing the following section, I was amazed at how open and honest she'd been and also impressed by her writing skills. At first, I wondered how to intersperse her paragraphs into the story, thinking that perhaps I would have them sporadically appear throughout, but upon reflection, I decided it would be most effective for you to read her passages verbatim.

. . . .

For nearly as long as I can remember, I have loved Andrew Dickin, so you could say I have been living my dream. I got the man I had wished for in my childish schoolgirl fantasies. But I hadn't bargained on him dragging his old friend Al with him. In the words of Princess Di "there were three of us in this relationship." In the heady rose-tinted flush of young love, I didn't realise his sneaky underhand little mate was tagging along for the ride, but sure enough, when I look back, he was always there, like the spectre at the feast, the unwelcome guest lurking in the shadows, ready to jump out and hijack the party.

I suppose I just thought, like everyone else, "well he enjoys a drink, everybody does it, he hasn't got a problem." And I should know, having spent a few years of my childhood with an alcoholic stepfather, the subject was one I had firsthand experience with. For the most part, I just let him get on with it. Yes, it caused rows from time to time, when he didn't want to leave a party, or he got that drunk he slept on the bathroom floor and we had to step over him to go to the loo in the night. How do you explain that to a small sleepy child? "Daddy thought he'd sleep on the bathroom floor in his undies, just for a change!"

The word 'alcoholic' can bring to mind the caricature image of someone on a park bench, swigging cider or surreptitiously sneaking drinks throughout the day without anyone knowing, or some lonely person in a bedsit with no money and no prospects. Andrew was none of those things. That's why people are so surprised when he tells them he's given up drinking. Everyone says, "WHY? You didn't have a problem and you weren't a real alcoholic!" He hid it well. It wasn't until he got older that it began to show in his appearance and health, and even then he got away with it because he was always at the gym or out on his bike, so everyone presumed he was fit.

For the last five years of Andrew and Al's friendship, he would wake up most mornings and tell me that was it, he wasn't going to drink again. "I've got to get a grip. I'm done with it, I want a healthy tea, no takeaways, no booze, I'll have a salad." I could almost set my watch by the phone call I'd get at 2.30pm in the afternoon, as his blood sugar was dropping and Al was wheedling his way back in. "I think we should have a Chinese tonight and some treats, just one last blast. I'll start next week." Eventually, I stopped being disappointed and just accepted that that was it – he always meant it but couldn't do it. On the rare weeks when he did actually manage to string a few good Al-free days together, then maybe my hopes were raised a little but, by weekend he was there, banging on the door of our lives, threatening havoc if we didn't let him in. Every time he told me he was serious about quitting, I jumped aboard the sober bus with him and clung on for dear life – it was always a bumpy ride. I attended doctor's appointments with him and hypnotherapy sessions and even reiki. I was with him when he went to see a counsellor. I made sure he took the pills that were supposed to get rid of his cravings. I supported him all the way. But nothing worked. Obviously, I became a little obsessed with trying to find a cure. I read lots of articles, joined forums and watched anything on TV regarding the subject. But when someone is hooked, they are hooked, and Al appeared to be winning the fight.

I think as the years passed, Al started coming between us more and more. Everything revolved around the next drink. If it was a bad day, it was a way to commiserate. If it was a good day, it was a way to celebrate, so there was always a reason. Even in the really bad days when money was tight and I was budgeting for everything, the wine and the beer still had to be bought, even if it meant borrowing off one of our boys. It's cringing to think about it now and I wonder why I didn't make a more forceful stand against it, but you can't win an argument with an addicted person. So I tried the subtle approach, like leaving articles about quitting open on the web browser or getting him to watch programmes about it. The thing was, he was in total denial about what it was doing to him. He'd stand in front of the mirror, drag his belly in and say he wasn't in bad nick for a man of his age and he'd talk about how fit he was on his bike and how many big hills he'd done. There's a lot of truth in the saying "there's none as blind as those who don't want to see." The sad thing was, I could see. I could see how the fit, agile young man I'd fallen in love with was disappearing right before my eyes. He was turning into a sweaty, bloated, middle-aged man who liked nothing more than getting his fill as fast as possible and falling into a comatose state in front of the TV. He wasn't great company, but at least I got the TV to myself after 7.30pm, as that was usually the time he'd be out of it by. I'd go to bed about 11pm and leave him laying there like a beached whale, snoring his head off. He'd usually crawl his way to bed a few hours later to wake up in the morning and pretend he didn't have a hangover. To be fair, he probably didn't most mornings because his body had grown used to the state, so nothing felt out of the ordinary. Sometimes, I would stare at him whilst he slept and wonder where and when it would all end.

Thankfully, I am not a drinker. I have the odd gin and tonic and maybe a Baileys at Christmas, but it really doesn't agree with me. I developed terrible migraines from my mid-twenties and if I had more than a couple of drinks, I paid a high price. Having said that, I did get a liking for red wine and that was because I would always pour myself one to prevent Andrew having a full bottle to himself. He would watch me like a hawk as I poured mine and I'd see the panic pass across his face if he thought I'd given myself too much. We used to laugh about it at the time, but to him it was serious. I was the boring one, the voice of reason, the nagging wife. But had I been like him and got the taste for it, I truly don't think that we would be here today. We would have drunk ourselves into oblivion. I think because I was there not wanting him to drink, it slowed him down and the one bottle of red a night never turned into two bottles. But then, he always had his beer.

The one trump card I always had up my sleeve was the calorie card. As the years passed and the weight crept on, every now and again, there would be a family do or a holiday to prepare for, and that's when Al would be banished to the naughty corner and I would take control (briefly). For a while, he would comply by limiting his intake, but it was always a very stressful time. The results were always short lived. Even though he felt better for it, Al always wormed his way back in. I knew that his weight was the one thing that concerned him more than anything else. He liked feeling slim, so he would wear the same comfortable pair of jeans and he didn't like me washing them too often because, as we all know, jeans do temporarily go a little tighter when newly washed. So I would wash and tumble dry them when he was out and put everything back in the pockets so he didn't know I'd done it and then when he put them on they felt tight. I know that's sneaky and underhanded, but I was desperate for him to get a grip before his health began to suffer.

One day whilst out walking, towards the end of Al's reign, we bumped into a friend we'd not seen for a while. She explained that she had not been well and although not much older than us and appearing quite fit, she had suffered a stroke. It turned out the headaches she'd been suffering were linked to her high blood pressure. She then went on to talk about drinking and how she'd had to cut down. As we walked away, Andrew told me he'd had a headache since his bike ride the day before and I could see what she had said was worrying him. As soon as we got home, he had me dig out my blood pressure monitor. The first time he used it, we thought it must be broken the reading was so high. So we decided to test the device on me. Lo and behold, my blood pressure was normal, so we did Andrew's again. The results were the same. High, and very alarming. We took his readings a few times that weekend and things didn't change, so Monday morning, he booked a doctor's appointment. I felt a huge surge of relief because all of a sudden, I had someone backing up what I had said. He was told he had to cut down and lose weight whilst not overdoing it with the exercise, and he had to really work at getting his blood pressure down as it was dangerously high. He did take this seriously and I think this was the starting point. He had been forced to think about his actions. So for a while he was on rations, one tiny individual glass bottle of red and two cans with one or two nights a week off. It helped, the readings improved, but they were still not good, and weekends still meant a binge party with Al up to his old tricks. During this time, Andrew was forced into the realisation that as hard as it was, there had to be a parting of the ways and it wouldn't be me that was sent packing, it was the villain of the story, Al.

I remember so well the day it all finally stopped. I think at the time I didn't believe that was it, as we'd been there so many times before and I'd given up hoping, but that cold bleak February day he stood before me with such a sad desperate look in his blood shot eyes, I hoped with all my heart that he could do it. We weren't in a good place financially and hadn't been for a long time. Plus, the weekend hangover that was still hovering and the fact that no money would be earned that week due to the severe weather, it all added to the feeling of desperation. Well, I don't need to go any further with what happened next, it's all written down in black and white.

As I write this little chapter, my very own tiny contribution to the story, we are nearly three years on from the tale of the beast and I can't believe the transformation. I am so proud of what Andrew has achieved and how things have turned around for us. I barely recognise the person he has become. The benefits are too many to mention and I am so grateful to him for facing his demons and booting them out the door, because I don't know where we would be right now if he hadn't. If I'd had to endure lockdown isolating with Al in the house, I just can't imagine the outcome. Who knows what the future holds at the moment for any of us, all I know is it's going to be better without the burden of the bottle.

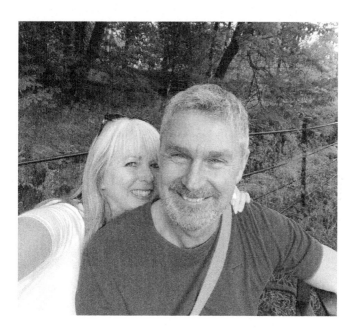

Chapter 6

Money Can't Buy Me Love

The immortal words of The Beatles, and how true they are. Money, indeed, can't buy you love – not true love anyway. It can, however, affect your life in innumerable other ways. I think Liza Manelli said it better; money makes the world go round. It is the fuel for everything (other than love) in this modern world of ours. We need shelter over our heads, so we part with our hard-earned money for that. We need fuel to get to our places of work, or maybe we use public transport, which also costs money. We do this to *earn* the money, to put back into travel once more. We use it to buy the food we consume, to *live*. Clothing, communication, entertainment, productivity, nourishment, the means to exercise; money has become the life-giver of the world in the 21st century. Some people don't have to worry about money. They have enough to do what they want, when they want, without giving it a second thought. On the other side of the coin, some people have to do backbreaking labour to just about afford to feed their families. They may eventually put enough aside to treat themselves, perhaps a short holiday, or a nice new pair of shoes, or maybe even a secondhand vehicle. Wherever you sit on the financial scales, life can drastically alter through the increase or decrease of your personal finances.

For somebody with an addiction, money almost takes on the form of vouchers. Tokens, fed into the machine in order to get the next fix. Payday rolls around, they check their bank balance, and they do this instant mathematics in their heads; "that will allow me to drink X number of beers this weekend" or "I can put X amount of this money on this football team tomorrow." Whatever the fix is, money is simply the means to fulfill it. Then, we have my Dad. Even if the amount of money in his bank *didn't* allow for X number of beers, or at least, it wouldn't leave him enough for anything else, he would still pump the tokens and get another hit of that oh so gratifying liquid.

By this point in his life, alcohol had become his key source of happiness. It was his ultimate escape from reality. Every night after work, he would head to the shops, fill up his basket of happiness, seat himself in his favoured spot on the sofa and begin the process of numbing himself against the trials and tribulations of life. Problems on a job? Drink. Argument with Christine? Drink. Loss of a loved one? Drink. No matter the issue, happiness will surely be at the bottom of this glass, or maybe the next one, or maybe this bottle of wine, or this bag of sweets, or this bag of peanuts!

But this escape comes at a price. For a family who has struggled to maintain financial stability from day one, flushing what little money we had down the toilet came at a cost that my Dad was not prepared for, one that would rob him of his business, would nearly leave our family homeless and himself alone, or maybe even worse. Due to his addiction our family faced possibly the most terrifying couple of years of our lives; terrified of somebody coming to repossess our belongings, or even to remove us from our home. And yet, through it all, my Dad continued to bury his head as far into the sand as possible. Daylight hours were spent worrying and depressed, desperate to come home and numb the pain. Once the intravenous was plugged in, everything was going to be ok, Andrew would tell us, in his delusional state of self-affliction. But of course, it wouldn't, not without drastic changes. And perhaps, with the experience we were about to face came a silver lining of its own; money became the key to my Dad's recovery. Of course, there were other straws putting weight on this camel's back, such as fitness and relationships, but when the penny quite literally dropped and the realisation came of what he was doing, my Dad realised that in order to fix the problem we faced, the booze had to go.

During our conversation for this chapter, we discussed how important this was. I said that I felt it was important because it was the lowest point of my Dad's drinking career. There are no funny stories to be told; no silver lining to be found. But not only that, that it was also the absolute embodiment of "the only way is up" when you've got as low as things got here. But my Dad disagreed on the latter point. He *did* agree that this was the ultimate low point for himself, but he states things could have got a lot worse, had he continued to live the way he was doing. He got a taste of what was to come, had things not changed, and it was absolutely terrifying. Enough for him to want to change things, but he could just have easily continued life as he was doing. After all, he believed it was his one true source of happiness!

．．．．．．．．．．．

1997 – Andrew was nearing the end of his time working at Preston's. He had experienced his dream job and had a good wage whilst doing it. He had learned valuable life lessons from his bosses that he still relies on to this day. Feeling the high life effect and with things looking good for our family, we decided to put our house on the market. We moved into a new home, still in Barnoldswick, and we still had some money left over from the sale. Life seemed to be moving along at a smooth pace. But in this state of happy days, the equity maintained in the house disappeared quickly on the pleasures of life, not least of which on Andrew's habit, a trend which would become incredibly prevalent in our lives. After leaving his job and having spent said money, the luxuries looked to be slowing down as quickly as they had sped up. But Andrew and Christine weren't ready for that and decided they wanted to take myself and my brother on our first foreign holiday, to Menorca. But of course, no money had been set aside for such endeavours, so how could we possibly afford that? In yet another trend that would manifest itself in Andrew, he decided to cash in an insurance policy, using the surrender value to afford the break. It goes without saying, we had an incredible family holiday, creating priceless memories and truly enjoying ourselves, but the notion of cashing in important things such as an insurance policy, simply for another dose of pleasure was one which Andrew would employ all too often from then onwards. He derived a new catchphrase for such occasions; "it'll be reyt."

But how did we go from the happy ending of the previous chapter to, once again, having no money and utilising cheap tricks to afford luxuries? Simple. Andrew's reluctance to not end the party was thriving. Having achieved his dream and feeling like a big player for having done so, he lived his life in a state of perpetual party, with his newfound slogan slapped right across his forehead. It was no longer a simple fact of wanting to be the last man standing at the soiree, it was now the need for every single evening to be his own private party. Takeaways, sweets, snacks and, of course, booze all became staple parts of his daily diet, spending at a much quicker rate than he could earn. He perhaps wasn't oblivious to how much he was spending, but the joy it brought him shone so brightly, he was blind to the future it spelled out for him and his family if he continued to expand his indulgent ways. The bank notes really did take on the form of alcohol coupons. He may leave for work in the morning with a £20 note in his pocket, but to him, that actually equated to £15/16 of happiness vouchers and a few quid left over to buy a cheap, petrol station sandwich, if he got hungry. And while he sat and gorged himself on his daily treats, all was right with the world. He would tell Christine his wild plans for sorting out issues; "I'm gonna ring so and so tomorrow, get that money he owes us" or "we should go on holiday, let's just sell sumert" – the high life is oh so alluring, especially when under the influence, when everything has an amber tinted glow. Of course, in the cold light of day, when he was hungover, depressed and anxious, he wouldn't ring so and so, he wouldn't sort anything out. He'd just spend the day thinking about the nighttime hours, when he could cast off his shroud of sense and responsibility and lose himself in the magical world of intoxication, where money worries don't exist and only happiness awaits.

We moved home, once again, in 2005. Staying in Barnoldswick, Andrew and Christine had found the perfect home for them and us. They were absolutely in love with the house and they felt like they had hit the jackpot in making it theirs. The high spirits experienced through the move dug their claws deep into Andrew's already rampant party status. This was *the* party house for Andrew, because he loved it so much, it felt like he was eternally on holiday, spending each night in a favoured villa. Except, he wasn't, of course. He was just digging himself further into his ever-growing hole. He recalls that after a year of living life this way, he found himself in my brother's bedroom one day, which from the window has a view of rolling hills, heading off into the beautiful countryside that surrounds our small town. As he looked out at the view, he started to question his actions, possibly for the first time. He found himself posing the question, in his head; "I wonder if I can keep this house?" He had finally acknowledged that the destructive lifestyle he was leading was surely unsustainable. Al approached and put an arm around his shoulder, peering out at the hills alongside him. "Don't worry about that, Andrew. Come on, let's go get tonight's goodies." And with that, this moment of clarity became shrouded, once more.

It was after this move, with this ceaseless party spirit now living in every fibre of Andrew's being, and within the walls of his home, that the daily "basketful of happiness" developed. Down the hill from our new home stands a petrol station, with a well-stocked alcohol section and an ample sweets aisle. Andrew would go there almost every evening and fill up a shopping basket with that evening's delights. He would fantasise about that moment all day whilst at work and felt an incredible buzz when the time came for him to drive down the hill and start picking off the shelves his supplies. He would enter the shop with a huge grin on his face, running a commentary in his mind to entertain himself as he goes, like he was playing some form of game show. Supermarket Sweep - Booze Edition. Or, if one of us had gone down with him, he would do it out loud. So high were his spirits, that his natural desire to be a clown came rushing to the surface in excitement, like a puppy who has just been told its feeding time. What would tonight's lager of choice be? I think we'll stick with Stella for tonight. Four pint cans thereof. Only the best! Now, wine, what are we having? This looks like a nice malbec. Oh, but hang on, it's only 12% ABV, that's no good. What about this one? 13.5%, that's better. It'll go down nicely with a load of peanuts and snacks. Speaking of which, don't forget them. A jumbo bag of salted will be perfect. Then we'll top the evening off with a couple of bags of sweets, maybe a box of chocolates too. Looking down at the contents of his basket was like looking into a world of bliss. No matter what was happening in the world around him, personal or on a larger scale, this basket was a solid guarantee of happiness. Everything was going to be A OK. Well, for 2 or 3 hours, at least, while it lasted. And when it was all over and Andrew dragged his assaulted body up to bed, he felt what he now refers to as F & F; fucked and full. The happiness tap had run dry and now the regret set in, feeling bloated, dizzy and refusing to look at himself in the mirror, to see the overweight, sad mess that would peer back at him from within. He got ready for bed in the dark, to ensure he wouldn't catch a glimpse.

By this time, Andrew had resumed his previous career as a decorator, having returned to the trade following his sidestep into the world of selling cars. He had started out on his own, having my brother, Chris, for an apprentice. As he started to take on more and more jobs, he became familiar with other local decorators, most of whom he befriended. They would recommend each other to possible clients and would help each other out where possible. Eventually, this coalesced into Andrew starting his own decorating firm, George Henry Decorators, named after his father and mentor, who had sadly passed away a couple of years prior. He continued to bring on more men to his team, with Paul "Snhoj" Johns as his right hand man. These were exciting times for Andrew. He had learnt staff management skills having analysed the workings of Richard and Simon Preston, as well as the managers of other car dealerships he had worked at, and the prospect of being able to take on so many jobs at once, sending out his various teams to different locations around the country was a very exciting one. And for a while, the business thrived. Through Andrew's incredible salesman techniques and with support from amazing friends, family and fellow businesspeople, he was able to establish an impressive portfolio of clients and contacts. He and his team decorate for the likes of Wayne Rooney, Steven Gerard, Katie Price, not to mention the impressive number of stately homes they would decorate on a regular basis. It seemed that the sky was the limit for the firm, with a boss who was a good laugh to work with and with a seemingly endless stream of high-end jobs. Andrew had successfully built up his business, but maintaining it was something else entirely, the rule book for which he refused to read.

It wasn't long until Andrew's tried and tested motto worked its way into the management of his business and some people started to take advantage of his laid-back nature. If he was owed money for a job, he wouldn't chase it up, or take any further action, other than to say, "it'll be reyt", living in belief that if he carried on as he was, it would eventually sort itself out. He counted the money he was owed as his, so he continued to spend as though he had already cashed the cheque. And then at the end of each day, he would drown his worries as usual, stating he was going to sort stuff out and the cycle would begin once more. Nothing would ever get sorted, it would just mount up until something gave way. It was inevitable that eventually this ramshackle tower, built on solid foundations and held up by good intentions would come crashing down, with a force that would eventually waken Andrew from his stupor.

Andrew received a letter one day, through the post. It stated that he owed money to the tax man. Of course, he didn't have the money, he was either owed it or he'd drunk it. But he didn't worry, he just continued to live unabated, sure that he would be paid the money he was owed soon, at which point, the bill could be paid. The weeks continued to roll on, with unpaid invoices mounting and more and more letters dropping through the letterbox. Yet Andrew still remained unperturbed. He continued to utilise his happiness basket daily, a means to numb himself and escape from the financial crisis that was rapidly coming upon him. And when he was sober, he was just as eager to find escape routes. He would ignore phone calls from numbers he didn't recognise. He would drive to nearby car parks, just to sit in his car, alone and not think about the situation, as much as possible. Now, it wasn't just his head in the sand, he was fully submerged, hoping that nobody but Al would find his hiding place. Christine was, naturally, very worried about the situation. Andrew wasn't telling her everything, out of reluctance to discuss the mounting problems, but Christine would see the letters coming through the door and knew he was ignoring them. Things looked bad on the surface, but they were even worse than they appeared.

Andrew was facing very dark days and it was starting to show not just internally, but externally, also. It was completely understandable why. He had very quickly gone from having a vastly expansive business with incredible prospects, an amazing team of workers who he considered to be very close friends and an amazing portfolio of work, to ignoring letters printed with the words "Do Not Ignore This Letter" because he could see the way the wind was blowing. It was, therefore, inevitable that these things would have an effect on Andrew. His standard of work started to slip, due to a lack of concentration. He started to realise he couldn't manage his team properly, having had no prior experience of such things and with the mounting financial concerns on top of that, things had just got completely out of hand, to an extent that Andrew simply could not maintain. He recalls working at a Premiership footballer's house, working hard to ensure the job was done to a high standard. His phone rang, meaning he had to get down from the ladder and answer it. It was the Inland Revenue, calling to discuss his ever-growing problems. What a bizarre situation to be in; decorating the house of a very wealthy person and having to interrupt his work to discuss his mounting money issues with the Inland Revenue. It was just all too much for him. The only thing he could do was to turn inwards, something unusual for a man who has spent his life as the life and soul of the party. Snhoj recalls that there was a three month period during which he didn't see Andrew once. And that went for the vast majority of his other employees, who would be going on jobs for a boss they had no sight or sound of for a long time. The fact was, with the growing pressure he was experiencing, he knew he couldn't face people. The thought of doing so filled him with incredible anxiety, to the point of sweating and panicking. In typical Andrew fashion, he assumed that if he could avoid his team seeing him in this way, they would continue to believe everything was ok, when in reality, it had the complete opposite effect.

Andrew used to attend a weekly business group meeting called BNI, Business Network International. In the glory days of his flourishing company, he loved attending these sessions, feeling like a big shot, rubbing shoulders with successful businessmen and being able to hold his own, reminiscent of his desire to hold his own with the old fellas at the Heifer. He would partake in the group sessions – delivering presentations on recent business successes and he relished in the possibility of earning new contacts, some of which led to the high calibre of jobs George Henry Decorators became known for. However, under the stresses of his current situation, Andrew began missing sessions, knowing that he couldn't put on the charade of the happy, bubbly person people of the group had come to know. The group cost somewhere in the region of £600 to join (which Andrew had charged to a credit card) and is run quite strictly, with a rule of being kicked out of the group for missing multiple sessions. Not wanting to attend in his current condition, but also worried about being removed from the group, Andrew called the chairman, Richard and explained to him that it wasn't that he didn't *want* to attend the meetings, it's that he felt he physically *couldn't* attend them. He told him that he didn't understand why, but he couldn't face people, the thought of which brought about incredible levels of anxiety. Richard, having dealt with endless businessmen, had heard this before and said, "it sounds like you might be going through a bit of a breakdown, Andrew."

Ruth, George Henry's accountant, was in our home office when Andrew returned home one day. She could tell straight away that he was behaving differently. He wasn't his usual loud, excited, happy self. She started to see a decline in him every time she came, like she was watching him slowly crumble. It began to upset her greatly to see him this way and upon leaving one day, she went to see another client of hers, Andrew Mclean, a good friend of Andrew's. Whilst there, they discussed my Dad's decline/breakdown, which had upset Ruth so much that Andrew had poured her a glass of wine to calm her down. Neither had ever seen him so despondent and seemingly detached. He was a shell of the man they both knew and cared for and it scared them to think that he might be losing his way, not to mention what that could mean for his and his family's future. They both concluded that Andrew needed help, so they contacted him and recommended that he go to the doctor's as soon as possible. He took their advice, now willing to admit that the problem had to be taken into his own hands, especially coming from people he respected as much as these two. Christine went along with him, of course, because she was incredibly concerned for his well being and wanted to make sure that whatever the doctor said, Andrew would follow up on. Afterall, it can be hard to pay attention to instructions when you are so trapped inside your own mind. The doctor diagnosed Andrew as depressed and prescribed him a course of antidepressants, which he would take from that day forward for 7 years, during which time, he continued to drink, despite the advice to not do so.

Eventually, Andrew decided to open one of the most recent letters, perhaps realising that they weren't going to end. Upon reading, he discovered that he owed £50,000 to the Inland Revenue, a figure that was incomprehensible to him. He was absolutely shellshocked to discover this. He had known things weren't good, but in his forlorn state, had simply looked the other way. This, however, was way worse than he initially imagined. He called Ruth, to see if she could explain. She told him that she had been trying to tell him for a long time and that by ignoring the issue, things had only gotten progressively worse. He couldn't wrap his head around the situation at all. He didn't understand how, in the space of a year, he had gone from being owed roughly £20,000 - £30,000 in unpaid invoices, to himself owing £50,000 to the tax man. His reluctance to follow the business rulebook had caught up with him and he didn't know which way to turn next, other than, of course, to run back to his basket, to continue to pretend things would eventually straighten out.

The following day, Andrew, hungover and facing a crisis, called the Citizens Advice Bureau, hoping somebody could help him out of the hole he'd dug himself into. He eventually ended up in an IVA situation, an 'Individual Voluntary Agreement'. Essentially, this is an agreement to payback what is owed to your debtors over an agreed upon length of time, designed to assist people in avoiding bankruptcy. These are the kind of situations that one may hear about but never expects to find themselves slap bang in the middle of, and this was certainly true of Andrew, who had thought the glory days of his business would never end. These were truly worrying times for him and Christine, that myself and Chris didn't really have a full grasp of (it is only now that I am writing this book that I myself actually know the full story of what happened during this period of Andrew's life). Following discussions with Ruth and others, Andrew entered into his IVA, with the terms laid out. He now had to work hard in order to meet these terms and to avoid a bankruptcy situation.

A year went by in this state. Andrew continued to utilise his basket to its full extent on a daily basis, spending his evenings numb and re-watching films with happy endings, in the vein hope that the joyous mood brought about from doing so would reflect on his own life and paint everyday life in brighter colours. The reality was that his desires were being swayed day after day by the temptations of Al and that the easy-to-obtain gratification that he could provide, instead of focusing his attention on the important things. The hole grew larger and larger, every time he filled up that basket.

In the Summer of 2012, Andrew arranged a belated "Christmas do" of sorts for the George Henry Decorators team. He took them to Alton Towers theme park for the day. He saw this as a chance to reconvene with his employees, who had seen less and less of him, and to have a full day of enjoyment, another form of escape from the harshness of reality. And it worked a charm, mostly. As soon as they arrived, Jason "Boo" Whalley got his face painted as a tiger, further solidifying the fact that he very strongly resembles Young Kenny from the TV comedy, Phoenix Nights. This served as a catalyst for the rest of the day, as they all laughed an incredible amount, with a high level of piss-taking going on between them all, all in good-nature of course. They all but forced the more nervous members of the team on to the most white-knuckle rides on offer, running around the park like a pack of excitable teenagers. Andrew actually describes it as one of the best days he's ever had, a strange thing to experience in the middle of one of the worst periods of his life. Towards the end of the day, things were starting to wind down. They had ridden all the rides, played enough games and were ready to slow things down a little, when they noticed a golf challenge, near the entrance to the park. The challenge was to get a hole in one, where the hole stood in the middle of a lake. Do so, and you could win yourself a car. They all decided to make it into a competition between themselves, seating themselves by the side of the lake and taking it in turns to go up and have an attempt. As this went on, some of them resigned and just sat chatting and laughing away, while Snhoj and a few others couldn't give up, refusing to be defeated by the challenge.

Whilst everyone was in high spirits from a truly delightful day, Andrew received a phone call from a number he didn't recognise. He stood up and walked away from the group, seated on the ground at the lakeside. It was a man calling from the VAT office. They were calling to inform Andrew that on Friday, 27th July, they would be doing a "drive by" repossession of all of the company vans. The vans that bore the name "George Henry – Decorators of Distinction" on the side. Losing these vans meant a lot. It was the beginning of the end for the company. Decorators need their vans, and with the name of the company – of which came from Andrew's beloved father – scrolled on the sides of them, it was as though the identity of the company itself was to be snatched away from him, all because of his own poor handling of a dire situation. As he stood with his back to the rest of them and received this devastating news, he began to cry, trying his best to hold himself together. This brief conversation had turned what had been, in his own words, "the best day ever", into a solemn celebration of the end. He ended the conversation taking on board the news he had received and tried to compose himself, drying away his tears discreetly and putting a fake smile back on his face in order to turn around and rejoin his employees, who were unaware of what Andrew had just learnt. Oblivious to the pain Andrew had just endured, they got back in the vans, the very ones that were to be repossessed in a matter of weeks, and drove home.

The day of the drive by came. It was a woman who came to see Andrew and to explain in detail how things were going to proceed. She started by reading him the "Riot Act." Partially listening, Andrew struggled to process the situation in his head. The whole thing felt completely surreal to him. He had no notion of these processes, or how to handle such things. He couldn't believe the situation he was facing. She informed him that the vans now belonged to them and gave him a date for the physical repossession of the vans, when people would come to actually take them away. She said if he was to sell the vans before this date, he would go to prison, yet another notion that Andrew struggled to process in his already tangled mind. When she had finished with all the legal processes necessary, she closed her book and said in a cheery way, "so, what are you doing tonight then? Having a glass of wine and watching the Olympics opening ceremony?", being the opening of the London 2012 Olympic games. He laughed to himself, thinking "*I can't believe what's going on here. I've let things get* this *bad and yet she asks if I'm going to have a drink and chill out tonight, almost like I'd be celebrating!*" But of course, almost like a clairvoyant, she was spot on, that is *exactly* what Andrew would do that evening. It was what he did every evening. Hide behind the bottle, away from the truth. But little did Andrew know, this was only the start of what was to come.

2013 – 2 years after its initial start, the IVA failed. Andrew had had numerous visits from officers from the VAT office, had spoken to departments he never imagined he would have to deal with, and the conclusion was that the Inland Revenue would be declaring Andrew bankrupt. A completely foreign concept to him, it would take a while for him to understand exactly what that means and what his next steps were for getting things in order. It's a scary word, bankruptcy. It conjures up images of empty bank accounts, living on the streets and even worse. His first step was to attend a meeting with the official receiver, to discuss what he had in terms of equity that could be used to pay off his debtors. Christine attended the meeting with him, but Andrew insisted she wear no jewelry or carry a nice handbag, or bring along anything that would show value, as they would likely note it down to be repossessed. Andrew claims he felt like he was living as a criminal, which was a very alien feeling for him. Following this meeting, Andrew was to arrange a trustee in bankruptcy and to come up with a settlement figure to be paid within 2 years in order to satisfy them. A trustee in bankruptcy will theoretically look after you through the bankruptcy process, handling your debtors and helping to relieve the financial strain you're facing. They're to collect the outstanding money owed to Andrew and are then to distribute it to his debtors on his behalf, while Andrew was to find the agreed upon figure. However, the trustees involved in Andrew's case advised Christine to also declare bankruptcy. This could have been avoided, but it was later discovered that it was advised because the mortgage on our home was in both their names and her declaring bankruptcy meant that if it came to ceasing the property, they could claim both shares of the mortgage fee, rather than just Andrew's half. She feels as though she was frightened into this position, being told that if anything was to happen to Andrew, his debts would then fall on to her. In reality, the money she owed on her credit cards was fairly insignificant, and in hindsight, could have been paid off, without her having to declare bankruptcy. I admit that this takes some wrapping your head around, or at least, it does for me personally, but essentially, this spells out that should the fee not be met after those 2 years, the house would be forfeit. Things were looking very real, for the first time and very desperate.

2 years slowly went by, with Andrew continuing to numb the pain. In his usual ways, he would continue his daily basket exercise, saying, "it'll be reyt", without really believing it but hoping everything would work out fine, despite the lack of a solid plan for conjuring up the money owed. Christine went through daily upset, fully believing that we would lose the house and our possessions. I remember discussions of where we would temporarily live, if it came to that. These were scary times. Eventually, time was up, and the money owed to the trustees had not been gathered. Which meant that Andrew was to go to court. He was given a date at Bradford court and he asked my brother to go along with him, as he didn't want to face it alone but also didn't want to put Christine through the whole ordeal. Chris agreed. Numbers were then flashed left, right and centre, with Andrew receiving advice from businesspeople he was close with as to how to handle the situation. He believed he had a strong defence for himself, with a settlement figure that he would present in court on the day. Having never experienced anything like it,

he had no idea how wrong he was to believe in his own defence like that. However, he convinced himself that he was in a strong position and that all would work out fine. As he sat there in the courthouse, waiting for his turn, the surrealness of the situation settled upon him once again. Where had he gone wrong in life? How had things gotten this bad? Could things have been different? When and how will all this end? As he sat and pondered these things, he was called in. Sweating and panicking, he stood before the judge and presented his figure, praying to all the gods that he would respond in kind. He thought to himself, "maybe the judge will see the state I am in, take pity and accept the figure." In reality, the judge shot him down, with an unchanged expression, delivered in the most dry, professional manner possible, the verdict was delivered that Andrew's offer had been declined. He was given 28 days to settle with his trustees, or the house became their property. Like taking a bullet in the chest at point blank range, Andrew was finished. Defeated. All possible avenues closed off to him. The gutter had its arms wrapped tightly around him, dragging him down into its depths. Despite the incredible mental anguish these events had lavished upon Andrew, a plan was formulated, that would mean we wouldn't become homeless. It would just take a little help.

． ． ． ． ． ． ． ． ． ． ．

I never understood any of this at the time of it happening. I knew things were bad and that my parents were attending meetings to do with finance, and I'd occasionally hear the words "bankruptcy" and "repossession", but I never knew the details until it came to talking to my Mum and Dad to write this chapter. I mentioned in my introduction that, unlike music and movies and TV shows, I never inherited drinking off my Dad. I would go out on a weekend when I turned 18 with friends, but that didn't last long, because that was around the time all this happened. Seeing how low my Dad was, both in terms of the things taking place and the mental condition he was suffering was enough for my young mind to be conditioned against drinking, through fear of my life following a similar trajectory. I remember when the notion of losing the house became a reality. I had gone for a walk with my Mum and the dogs. She was very quiet, which is unusual, as we often talk about a lot of things when we're out for a walk. I asked her what was up and she loosely explained to me that within the year, unless a miracle was to occur, we would lose the house. Of course, this was a very pessimistic viewpoint from her, and we didn't lose the house, despite no divine intervention, but I began to understand the anguish she was going through. It changed my approach to speaking to my Mum and Dad during this time, as I was worried to learn more. I suppose, like my Dad, I wanted to pretend none of it was happening. I would be sat watching television on an evening with my Mum and an intoxicated father, when a car – or even worse, a van – they didn't recognise would pull onto the street. You could feel the atmosphere in the room change instantly as they thought it was someone coming to start repossessing our belongings. This went on for years, even after the event, in a post-traumatic way. Even now, to this very day, they still get shifty about it, especially if the person behind the wheel is in a suit, looking all official. The lasting effects it had on the minds of both of them and, to an extent, on me and Chris too, is extraordinary, especially to think that in a very real sense, it all stemmed from Andrew and his escapism, facilitated by Al.

A Sobering Thought

The Apple Doesn't Fall Far from the Tree

Christopher Dickin, my brother, is just like my Dad in many ways. He has inherited from him the natural ability to be incredibly irritating 98% of the time. It is actually impressive, at times, just how naturally he hits upon something maddening, and how long he manages to keep it up. I remember one time being in his van, driving into town to pick up a takeaway. From the second we got seated in the van until we stepped back through the front door at home, he *screamed* the same thing, endlessly – "88 miles per hour! 68 miles to the gallon." There was no rhyme or reason for him to do this, only to attempt to drive me to despair. After years of watching our Daddy dearest doing things of a similar nature, I suppose it rubbed off on him. And even now, just as he is about to hit 30 years old, people think I am the older brother. I suppose I, too, can be irritating at times, I'm sure my partner, Charlotte, would confess to that, so I can't say that that particular quirk of my Dad's skipped a generation with yours truly. But one gene I didn't inherit was the Al gene. Chris, on the other hand, says that he did.

I wanted to ask Chris some questions, to see how he felt about our Dad's decision to never drink again, what his own personal relationship with drinking is and whether he felt an influence from Andrew's habits. I video called him and pressed record on my phone. He started out talking in an American accent, he farted a few times throughout, he occasionally made random yelling noises, but the answers he gave me were truthful, despite some nonsense and my Dad, upon listening to his responses, could see himself reflected in the answers throughout, understanding the mindset that Chris has.

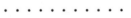

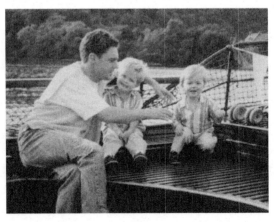

Jonny: Ok, question one.

Chris: (American accent) Yeah, okay, sure. Hit me with it.

J: Do you think Dad had a problem with alcohol?

C: Yes. I do. (mercifully, he dropped the accent here) Because he couldn't not have a drink. And, on the way home from work (*Chris is a decorator too, and would often work with Andrew*)... in a morning he would say he was done with it and on the way home, he'd buy some cans, which to me says that he's really battling something there. He was fighting against what he clearly knew was right and what he knew wasn't, kind of thing.

J: Do you think his problem could be passed on to either you or me?

C: (*Laughs*) Yes. Yes, I do.

J: Do you want to elaborate at all?

C: Well, I think I've got it.

J: Right, and do you think that's because you saw him and his problem?

C: I don't know about that, because, maybe subconsciously it did, but all my mates were doing it, so I did it too. Every single one of my friends did it, and did it before I did. So, I suppose I was just joining in. And then that turned into getting cans in at home [not just drinking socially]. So maybe it was subconscious, since I'd seen that go on all my life.

J: But when you say that you'd get cans in at home, do you think that was because that's what Dad did?

C: Yeah, I think so, because a lot of my mates didn't really do that bit, but I just thought that was what you were supposed to do. I think growing up on building sites added to it a lot, because they all do it. They all stop and get cans on the way home from work.

J: What do you think of the fact that Dad hasn't had a drink in so long?

C: I think it's good, I want to do it.

J: You want to do it? Stop drinking?

C: Yes, and I'm going to do it.
J: Do you think it's impressive?

C: Yes, I do, and I think everybody you talk to about it wants to do it, too. Everyone you talk to – even if they're the one to ask you about it – because when I gave up for a while before, people would say "are you having a drink?" and I'd say "no, I don't drink", they instantly go on the defensive, as though I were telling them not to [have a drink]. But, obviously, I wasn't, but they'd be like "well, I only have two or three of an evening." So, yeah, I think everyone wants to do it really.

J: So you think that engaging someone in a conversation in the subject can put their defenses up if they're not willing to admit that they'd like to stop, too?

C: Yes, I do. Because I've been there and done it myself.

J: Do you ever think about Dad's problem when you're drinking, or when you're suffering from a hangover?

C: I'm not sure I know the answer to that question.

J: Well, say like this weekend for example, you've not been well (*after a couple nights of binge drinking*). Has it crossed your mind that you don't want to do the same things as Dad in

terms of addiction, or that you *do* want to do the same as him in terms of quitting?

C: I want to do what he's done [quit drinking] but a lot sooner in my life than he did. And yes, that has crossed my mind while I've been hungover this weekend.

J: But it doesn't cross your mind when you're drinking?

C: No, no, at the time, it makes sense. If I were to stop and think about it while drinking, I'm not going to enjoy myself, and that's a reason for drinking, so I'll just put it out of my mind until the morning. I think about it a lot at work, too.

J: I don't want to put words into your mouth, but when we were young, did you look at Dad drinking and think "I want to do that, too?"

C: Urm, yeah, a bit. I don't know what it was about it, but it appealed to me. I'm not sure why, but it was like, well Dad would have cans with his Sunday lunch or whatever and then he'd get all silly, and what have you, and then I'd just think that it looked like good fun. And also, whenever anybody talked about it, they'd talk about good, fun times, you know. So, everything about it appealed to me.

J: Yeah, well, I remember telling Dad that when we were younger and we'd be visiting Grandad Adrian, you'd have a taste of Grandad's beer and you'd be telling yourself that you liked the taste. Do you think that was because you actually *wanted* to like it?

C: Yeah, because all the blokes were doing it. I remember pinching a beer of Dad's when I was young and sitting on the stairs and drinking half of it and he went mad at me.

J: (*laughs*) Really? I don't remember that! How old were you?

C: I'm not sure, but we lived at Sycamore Way (*our house which we left when Chris was 13*). It was around the time I put salt in his beer, do you remember that?

J: (*laughs*) No, not at all!

C: Yeah, we'd sat down to Sunday lunch and his beer was on the table before he arrived and I put *loads* of salt in his beer because he'd bollocked me for something earlier. He went fucking apeshit and

141

now when I think back, I understand why, because every can mattered, because he weren't going to be going back out to get some more.

J: Did you see drinking as a tradition you wanted to continue?

C: I think, because it wasn't that much of a big deal, that I didn't think the kind of things you're asking me in these questions. Because it just wasn't a big deal. I just saw it as something that everyone did. I never thought "oh I need to carry that on", I just thought well I'll just do the same. I don't know. I wasn't thinking Grandad drank and Dad drinks, so I will too. It was just what people did when they got to that age.

J: Yeah, I see what you're saying. The reason I ask that is because when Dad was younger, he used to watch his Dad and his friends drinking and actually aspired to do the same thing. Was it not the same for you?

C: Yeah, I know. But he was down at the Heifer (*the pub*) and watched them drinking and that, whereas Dad didn't. We just watched him drinking at home and falling asleep on the sofa, so that was the normal thing. But obviously, when we were younger, I didn't realise it as a problem and by the time I did and I realised he was slurring his words and stuff, I was already drinking. I mean, I used to tell him to not drink, for Mum's sake, but at the same time, I was doing it.

J: I know what you mean. I said in the Introduction that when I was younger, I didn't think of it as anything out of the ordinary, I just thought that all Dads drank every night like he did.

C: Yeah, exactly, adults have beer and it's as simple as that. We used to leave cans of Stella out for Santa on Christmas Eve. Even when I knew Santa didn't exist, the cans were still getting drunk.

J: Oh right, so... Santa didn't have it?

C: No, no. Dad had it.

J: Ahh, right, because it's traditionally milk isn't it?

C: (*laughs*) Yeah, traditionally.

J: Do you ever wish that you would stay sober for the rest of your life?

C: Yeah. If someone said to me now, you can go sober and you won't... Actually it's a hard question to answer, because it's the not wanting a drink that I want. I can be sober for the rest of my life, but if it never goes away that I want a drink, I'll be pissed off.

J: But that's something that has never gone away for Dad either. He doesn't crave it every day, but it does still strike him every now and then.

C: Yeah, I know. And I had those feelings when I stopped drinking for 7 months earlier this year. I'd like to be able to do like Olivia (*Chris's partner*) and just have one or two a night if I fancy it. But if somebody said to me that I can flick a switch now and be sober for the rest of my life and not be bothered by it, then of course I would.

J: Do you think you could ever be at a point where you can just have one or two, does it have to be all or nothing, like Dad?

C: It's all or nothing. Maybe when I'm older and I've got kids or whatever then I might be different, it's hard to say. But to be honest, I like the all or nothing. If I'm a drinker, I'm a drinker. But if I'm not drinking, I like to be able to say that I'm not. If somebody asks me if I like a drink, I like to be able to say that I don't, because not everyone can do that. But if I'm only having a couple, then I have to say well, yeah, I do. It's not worth it. You're being either hung for a sheep or a lamb, or whatever they say.

J: You might as well be hanged for a sheep as for a lamb.

C: Yeah, or whatever it is. If I'm drinking, then I'm drinking. But I'd like to be able to say that I don't.

J: Is there anything else you'd like to say?

C: It's a problem for me [drinking], but nearly all my mates drink as much as I do, and to the extent that I do. There's only a select few that don't. I don't necessarily see what I've done as anything noteworthy. But because it's been built up so much by Mum and Dad, you know, Mum always told me that I shouldn't drink as much as I do, I've always seen it as a problem. I don't regret that I've been a drinker, I've had a lot of fun doing it. But it led me to the point of thinking about stopping. There are some people my age who have never drunk, but they might start later in their life, whereas I've already done it now.

. . . .

I think what Chris was trying to say was that he has learnt through his experiences. He has enjoyed his time drinking, made good friends and been to many places and done many things, but that he would now like to put it behind him, which is, obviously, easier said than done. He mentioned how he has had extended periods of not drinking, but he has started up again every time, and he talks about how that want for a drink never goes away. It would be a lie to say that quitting was easy, and those cravings are just one of the hurdles that can bring an end to a sobriety period. But those challenges must be faced down in order to achieve that goal, if that is what you truly want. If you want the rainbow, you've got to put up with the rain.

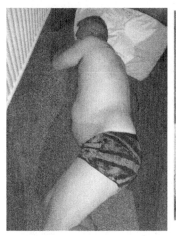
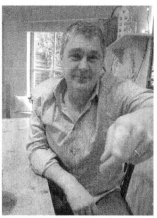
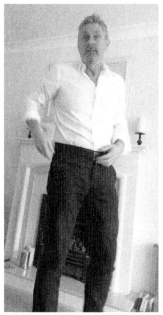
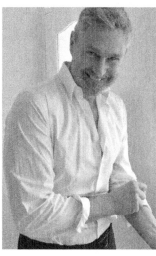

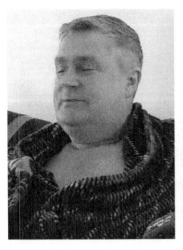
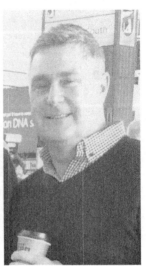
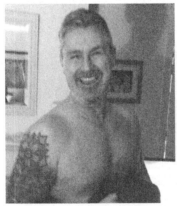
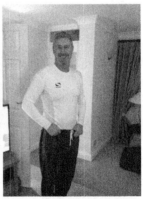

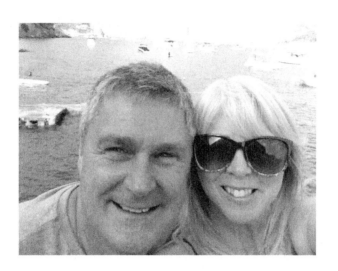

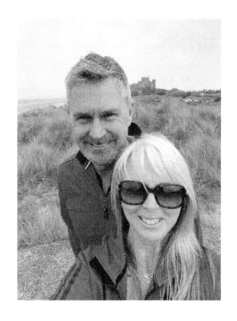

Chapter 7

A Little Help from my Friends

The vessel seemed all but doomed, as more and more water billowed through the large gaps in the hull, submerging everything inside with the dark, unforgiving waters of the vast ocean, of which they had once set out upon, brimming with pride, glory and elation. Over the years, the ship had faced incredible hardships: enormous waves, sea monsters taken straight from a Herman Melville novel, thunderstorms that would put the frighteners up Poseidon himself, but it had faced down each one, turning to avoid collision with such treacherous events. However, years of close calls had left the ship in a rundown condition. Cracks had begun to form on its outer casing, its mast was beaten and worn from overuse and in their overtired state, the crew members had grown lax to problems that could have easily been avoided through a little foresight and course correcting.

The trials and tribulations of the vessel had all been heralded by the ship's captain, who maintained that there were no issues to speak of, that if they continued unabated on their current course, the future held nothing but triumph and unimagined riches. His crew would try their best to warn him of the tragedy that lay on the horizon; the fact that after years of maintaining his craft, it may soon lay at the bottom of the ocean, all of them trapped within, sealed in a dark, drowned coffin. But the blame cannot be put upon the captain's shoulders alone. For you see, he had a first mate. Someone who would shower him with praise, fill him with emotions of joy and ecstasy, overall leading him to believe he could do no wrong. "Stick with me, Captain. Those others don't know what they're talking about. This ship has sailed for years now and will sail for many more to come. A few waves and thunderstorms aren't going to stick us!" Blinded by his first mate's flattery, the captain believed every word spoken, and so continued his course, making no adjustments or fixes.

Then came the day. With the ship skipping across the water, the captain fixated on his goal and his crew doing all they could, the ship sprung a leak. The cracks in the outer casing could hold no more, and the aforementioned billowing in of the water began. The crew sprang to attention, alerting the captain of the issue and trying their best to formulate a plan that could save them from the inevitable doom. But try as they might, with the captain providing no aid, continuing to bask in his first mate's adulation, it seemed this was the end of their voyage.

Just as all seemed lost, with the crew crippling themselves to bail water out of the ill-fated ship, two crew members stepped forward, with a plan that could put them back into a state of smooth sailing, onwards towards the goal of exultation. They revealed to the captain that they had brought along a private bundle of supplies, which they were saving for use at a later date. One of the pair had even borrowed the supplies from an onshore loaner, with the promise of a larger return in the future. The pair informed the captain that they were willing to give to him and the rest of the crew their supplies, in the hope that it would be enough to patch up this increasingly alarming situation. The captain, now aware of the severity of the proceedings, accepted the bounty incredibly graciously, assuring them that he would return the favour in kind once things were proceeding smoothly once again. He rallied his crew, handed out the supplies and they sprung straight to action, repairing the holes, bailing the remaining water and allowing the ship to correct itself, standing upright on the surface of the water, pointing dead ahead, towards its goal. The captain was elated. He expressed his enormous gratitude to the pair and his crew, who had saved him from a certain watery grave.

At the end of this long, trying day, the captain retired to his quarters, where he sat in his favourite chair, to ponder what he now must do to maintain his vessel and ensure that nothing of this sort could ever happen again. As he relaxed into his seat, his first mate stepped forward from the shadows, a grin across his face. He had been nowhere to be seen during the day, as all others on board worked tirelessly. Yet here he was now, ready to lather the captain with his adulation, once again.

For the next few weeks, nobody saw the captain or the first mate. They remained locked away in his quarters, laughing and joking, drinking and smoking - blissfully unaware that his once beloved vessel was decaying, yet again, and that it would not be long before disaster came knocking upon the hull once again.

. . . .

Andrew would never forget that day in court, with his eldest son by his side, contemplating the wrong choices and actions that had led him there. The moment the judge declared that he was to lose his home in a month's time would haunt him for the rest of his life. Who could have possibly imagined that those carefree days of longing to be a drinker would lead to this outcome? Drinking just looked like fun to him. It was the thing that "men" did. It's what "men" are "supposed" to do. But why had nobody told him that it could have such devastating results? Or, maybe, in actuality, it was time to face facts, to admit people had warned him right throughout his life, that he had ignored the warning signs, blinded by his life's fuel. Or at least, when people started to see the change in Andrew, from a slim, athletic, calm and collected man into an overweight, sweaty, anxious man with high blood pressure, people (Christine, in particular) started to express worry that it would leave him with nothing, maybe even cost him his life. And now, there he stood. He had blown past the warning signs a long time ago. They were many miles back south. The reality that faced him now was the one in which they had foretold. 28 days until sundown.

Andrew and Christine had little to no time to dwell on the emotional impact of the outcome, instead they had no choice remaining but to get their heads together and to think about the physicality of the situation. Where would we live once our home was repossessed? We couldn't afford a new home (of course not, otherwise we would have just paid the money owed to stay put), and so options were thrown around of going to live with relatives, such as Andrew's Mum, Shirley, in her small home in Kelbrook, back in Andrew's childhood bedroom. These conversations would leave Christine distraught. She had loved her current home more than any she had ever lived in. The thought of one day, in the not-to-distant future, driving by the house and seeing somebody else inside; somebody sat in *our* living room, cooking food in *our* kitchen, sleeping in *our* bedrooms was enough to drive Christine to tears, and although Andrew tried to maintain that everything would work out in the end, he himself would feel the same way, mortified that the home he had worked hard to maintain would belong to someone else. But the options were severely limited, and time was swiftly running out. The ship was sinking. Just as all seemed lost, two individuals took it upon themselves to be our saving grace.

Andrew needed to come up with £30,000 to save the house, an impossibility. He couldn't take a loan out, the banks and lenders wouldn't go near him and any money he had had was long gone, flushed down the toilet after an evening with Al. But that didn't mean somebody else in the family couldn't take a loan out. The responsibility fell to Chris. My brother and I had lent money to my parents before, at desperate times, or occasionally for less important things, i.e.: booze. But this was way above and beyond a simple lend. After discussing the possibility and with the deadline looming, Chris agreed to take out a loan of £15,000, getting Andrew halfway to his target. Andrew and Christine would deal with the monthly repayments, transferring Chris the required amount each month to cover the loan, plus the interest. Of course, this is a lot to ask of a young man in his early 20's, but desperate times call for desperate measures. The other half came from an incredibly generous and kindhearted friend of Andrew's, who simply wanted to see him back on his feet and to see him succeed and be the person he once was again. He told Andrew to not worry about getting the money back to him in any rush and to just concentrate on getting back on the straight and narrow. An unimaginable gesture from a friend, alongside Chris's loan, was the structural support that Andrew needed. We were able to keep the house, an eventuality thought inconceivable. The ship had been saved from going under, it was time to point it in the right direction and ensure it stays afloat.

With the house saved, the focus became getting together the money owed to both Chris and Andrew's friend. Time was more on our side now. It couldn't wait forever, but the weight of a 28-day time limit now alleviated, some of the pressure had been released. This was both a blessing and curse, as you shall soon see.

A fall from grace such as the one Andrew had suffered came with some consequences of a certain nature, that being that he felt embarrassed about what he had gone through, and having to admit the reality to friends and family was crushing for him. Not only that, but the anxiety induced by an unknown car driving down the cul-de-sac, even after the case was settled, remained. They found they were struggling to relax and be comfortable in their own home. Now seemed as good a time as any to cut and run, make a fresh start somewhere else. As much as they had fought to keep the house, the logical solution was to now sell it, hopefully netting them enough money to pay back both loans and have enough left to either start up afresh in a rented house, or to downsize. Whichever it may be, the idea was that it wouldn't be in Barnoldswick. The pair pondered where they could move to: the Lake District, Northumberland, Majorca was even tossed around as an idea. It was a strange mix of emotions. They would be walking away from their beloved home, but it was also a chance for something new and exciting. They could leave the past where it was. But before they could run, they had to walk, which meant they first needed to get the house sold, a task which came with its own set of problems.

Following Andrew's bankruptcy, with the looming possibility of a home repossession, Andrew and Christine took an unusual tack; they let their home become somewhat run down. Rooms were left undecorated for a long time, roof tiles were left out of position, leaks were handled with nothing more than a bucket underneath them and so on. This was in the vain hope that, should it come to it, which of course it did, the house would be valued lower than it could have been had it been in mint condition, therefore making the settlement figure lower. It seems crazy to think that my parents could actually conceive of such a plan, but, as I have already stated, desperation can lead to some unexpected decisions. Who's to say whether this plan worked or not, for we can't see an alternate reality, in which the house was in pristine condition and was subsequently valued higher, meaning we were unable to keep it, but in actuality, it left us with the issue of having a rundown house, which we now needed to sell. In order to do so, the house would require a lot of care and attention, which requires money and time; two things Andrew had proved to be no expert at handling. In order to get the house up to scratch, Andrew was going to have to take some time off work. But he couldn't. We were skint, so we needed him to work as much as possible, to bring in enough to pay back the loan. It was a complete Catch 22 situation. And so, in typical Andrew Dickin fashion, he said "well, we'll stay here until after Christmas, get some money behind us, then we'll do it up, get it on't market and move on." So that was the new plan. Enjoy the time we have left here, because come January, the cogs will be in motion. Christmas was upon us in no time, money remained sparse, and what little we had was spent on Andrew's favourite hobby, Christmas being Andrew's ultimate binge period. January came next, and there was no sign that Andrew would be taking any time off to concentrate on the house. "Be reyt, I'll get on it in't next few weeks or so." This trend continued for a long time. Each week would come the conversation of just *when* the work would start on the house. Before we knew where we were, another Christmas had passed us by, another year in the history books, and yet we remained unmoved. Need I state *why* money was sparse, *why* we hadn't moved forward at all? It had nothing to do with a shortage of work; Andrew remained as busy as ever, working every day (by now, mostly on his own). It was, of course, Al and his basket.

Instead of learning from his mistakes, counting his blessings that, with a little help from his friends, things could get back on track (don't get me wrong, his gratitude for such assistance has never been in question), he relied even more on Al, a friend who would only lead him back to that dark, dank place he had not so long since escaped from. Andrew claims that this period was his worst for his reliance on his basket, which makes sense, given the wounds inflicted by the whole ordeal and the fact that he truly believed that drinking was the only medication for such wounds. But it left us, once again, trapped in a loop. How could we ever save up money if we're just earning enough to pay Chris *and* buy the nightly basket?

The reason for this increased reliance on the cherished basket was the new veneer cast over Andrew by the preceding events; he became an angry, bitter man. As though there was somebody to blame, perhaps the global cosmos, the wealthy elite, whatever it was, fault would not be accepted by him. He couldn't see clearly, couldn't understand that it was his own issues that had led us to where it had and if that thought did cross his mind, he had to convince himself the fault laid elsewhere, an argument in his own mind, facilitated by the drink. He argued with people he loved. He fell out with fellow decorators, who he had spent years working day-in-day-out with, he shouted at events happening on the television, as though they could hear him. Overall, he became an unpleasant person to be around when in this state, unrecognisable from the happy-go-lucky, soul of the party Andrew he once was. And so, in light of this newfound bitterness, he would rely on his basket even more in the knowledge that it was a guaranteed source of happiness after a day of anger and frustration. Unless he could get these complicated emotions under control, they were indicating that we would end up back in the gutter, after being clutched from his grasp at such a desperate time.

There was another element caught up in this Catch 22: Andrew's physical condition. By this point, he was the heaviest he had ever been, had more chins than he'd ever had and had resorted to living in elasticated waistbands and black tops, because everyone knows they're slimming. Unfortunately for Andrew, that only works to a point, and it was becoming increasingly difficult to hide his inflated torso. The embarrassment, anger and frustration caused by his appearance had a familiar cure: the basket. Like all other issues in his life, Andrew sought refuge in his daily happiness source. But of course, this only made the situation worse, a reality Andrew could care less about when he had a can of lager in one hand and the other reaching into a bowl of mixed peanuts. Half a bag of salted, half a bag of dry roasted. And once he'd railed his way through those, reluctantly eaten the meal Christine had prepared (reluctance being the result of having less of an appetite following the nuts), then came the sweets and chocolates. Full, sharing bags of fruit pastilles, entire bars of Cadbury's Fruit and Nut (at least the raisins were one of his five a day!). This daily diet really was seen as a form of medicine to him. He recalls now how ludicrous it is that such a thing could bring him such enormous pleasure. An obscene amount of salty/sugary snacks, alongside his daily alcohol intake was doing incredible damage to him and the thought of such a thing now, in hindsight, is baffling to him. Back then though, he told himself that, being past the age of 50, come hell or high water, this is what he is now. It's too late to change things. Much like the sentiment he had when Christine first raised the flag on his drinking back in their youth, he stood his ground. This is the way things are, like it or lump it.

With a glaring problem such as the one Andrew had, we bumbled along for a long time, what little money left over after the loan repayments being squandered. We couldn't save any money in case we ended up back at the bottom and Andrew couldn't afford time off. His health was a risk to his life and wellbeing, his relationships with people were diminishing due to his own negativity, his happy times came only through the cost of more weight gain and money loss... things looked just as dire as before, only this time, it was much more personal for Andrew, and we could all see it happening before our very eyes. Everything taken into consideration, it was clear nothing was going to be accomplished, and whichever way we looked at things, it was all a result of Andrew's addiction. He had been pulled out of the quicksand by some incredibly considerate people, only to not step off it through the advice of Al. Things were so bad that, had they accomplished the task of selling the house, Christine intended to hide the remaining money away from Andrew for fear that if he got his hands on it, it wouldn't be long before it was all pissed away once again. She never imagined that she would even have to consider such a thing in the early days. That her husband would become so enamored with drink that she would have to physically hide funds away from him, for his and her own good. The craziest part is this was actually Andrew's idea. In a real Jekyll and Hyde moment, Andrew saw clarity and realised that his greed would take over and that it would be out of his control, and so he would have to make plans against himself, through the aid of Christine. Needless to say, this is not a healthy way to live. There was only one way out of this never-ending loop, and that was for him to give up the drink altogether, a task that is much easier for me to write and for you to read, than it is for a person such as Andrew Dickin to achieve.

Chapter 8

Three Wheels on my Wagon

I'm pretty confident in saying most people who drink on a regular basis have, at some point or another, woken up after a heavy night on the booze and said, "never again." Suffering from chronic headaches, throwing up, loss of appetite…. hangovers are dreadful. Personally, I rarely drink. Besides the obvious reasons for not doing so, I tend to suffer from serious hangovers the day after. Maybe it's my body's way of telling me to not follow my Dad's footsteps. I remember waking up on the floor of a friend's bedroom one New Year's Day. I slowly started to open my eyes when, all of a sudden, a beam of light, just barely creeping through from under the Velux blind caught my eye and it felt as though a steam train had made firm contact with my forehead. At that precise moment, memories of the night before - which, I'd enjoyed, maybe a little too much - came flooding back to me, not least of which just how much alcohol I had consumed. Up until that point, I had drunk on a fairly regular basis. Nothing that could be considered close to a problem, but I would go to the pub most weekends with my friends, spend lots, drink lots and wake up feeling worse for wear the day after. But from that particular morning forward, when my brain collided with the Flying Scotsman, drinking sessions became few and far between. I had properly experienced how painful a hangover could be, as I spent the rest of the day hardly being able to keep down a small glass of water. That was enough for me to know I had reached my limit.

My Dad, as you know by now, would wake up in those states, occasionally (he obviously had a much higher tolerance for these things than I did), say "never again" and then would be supping down some Stella later that day. His relationship with drinking was much more deeply rooted than mine, and breaking it off isn't as easy as saying "I'm done with drinking" and that's it, end of. It's like a complicated, love/hate relationship that's very difficult to find the correct route out of.

The other issue he faces is that for him, it's all or nothing. He carries that quality in all facets of his life and so of course it applies to his, at the time, number one hobby of drinking. He couldn't just cut down to a couple of times a week, or fewer cans of an evening. If he's drinking, he's having the lot. If he's cutting down, he's stopping. There is no middle ground.

For me to document every attempt my Dad made to give up would require a whole other tome. Granted, most of the entries would be "gave up on Monday, started drinking again on Tuesday," but the number of entries would be endless. But there were three attempts at "getting on the wagon", as they say, that stand out in Andrew's drinking career, where it seemed like the light at the end of the tunnel was drawing near.

"... And I'm still rolling along"

. . . .

July 2011 - Andrew had made one of his all too familiar proclamations. He was done with drinking. It was greeted by everyone with the usual levels of apprehension and we all expected that within the next 24 hours at some point, he would be occupying his favoured living room spot with Al, intoxicated once again. A week went by and he hadn't touched the stuff. Still, he'd done that before, but it was impossible to not feel a little pride, which I'm sure he felt within himself too. He had decided that it was time to face facts with regards to his weight. He longed to be the slim, athletic man he once was, believing it wasn't too late to turn things around. He started running, something he had passionately done as a young man, he was eating healthy, home cooked meals, his bike rides felt easier and the weight slowly started to dwindle. He passed the 2-week mark, then 3, 4... A month with no drink. It seemed incomprehensible, but he was proving us all wrong.

Andrew and Christine went away for a short break in Northumberland, staying in a small cottage next to Bamburgh beach, their favourite place in the UK. They took our two dogs with them for a week-long holiday of walking and sightseeing. Naturally, Christine was nervous about the holiday, as that was prime bonding time for Andrew and Al, as they would usually party the week away. But, rather incredibly, the week went by without so much as a sniff of booze. Rather, Andrew continued to exercise, rising early in the morning, putting on his running shoes and going down to the beach for an hour's run along the coast, as the brisk, Northumberland air revitalised his lungs. Perhaps he was a changed man? It certainly seemed that way, as he had never achieved a month without drinking. It was completely unheard of. But he breezed past it, with an incredible amount of pride encouraging him to stay seated on his wagon, billowing along at a pace Al couldn't match.

Around this time, Andrew prepared to head down south with Snhoj to work on a big job they had acquired through a new client. They were to decorate the home of Katie Price, AKA, Jordan. This meant that they would be staying away from home for roughly 6 weeks, depending on how long the job would take them to complete. Snhoj, being a lot younger than Andrew and enjoying the things younger people enjoy - such as going out to clubs and bars - would likely have made the most of being away from home and in a new town, sourcing out the best drinking spots and painting the town red. Instead, in solidarity with his friend, he decided that he would join Andrew in not drinking for the time they were there.

It didn't take long, however, for temptation to sneak in for Andrew. They set off on the long journey down to Sussex on the August bank holiday weekend. The weather was glorious, casting a blanket of heat over the pair as they traveled down. They called at Lymm Services for a break when they noticed lots of people caked in mud and neon face paint. "Bet they've been at Creamfields," Snhoj worked out as they walked into McDonalds. As Andrew saw these young people, who had spent the weekend in the sun, partying, under the influence, he felt a surge of jealousy. Not necessarily for the musical acts they had experienced, more for the fact they had spent the weekend intoxicated in the beautiful southern weather. The craving for a long, cold beer was massive. But he resisted. They ate their burgers and fries, drank a cold drink apiece and got back in the van to continue their journey.

The long journey came to an end as they reached their new, temporary home of Horsham. They checked into their Travelodge, swiftly unpacked, each had a shower and then headed into the town to get a feel for where they would be living for a while, and also to find somewhere to eat. They eventually settled on Pizza Express. While sat there, eating pizza and sipping a Diet Coke, Andrew could see everyone else pouring back large bottles of Italian lager. This was his first real test. He didn't have his wife by his side to discourage him, though he did have a close friend, who I suppose was his acting wife during this time. But still, seeing how easy these bottles were going down for everyone else was like torture for him. He could see Al moving from table to table, opening bottles for people, pouring them into a cold glass with just the right amount of head, all the time trying to lull Andrew in, tempting him more and more with each release of a bottle cap. With the bait luring him in, Andrew picked up the menu, to see how much a bottle of the golden fluid would set him back. His Yorkshireman roots came rushing to the surface at the sight of a £6 price tag. And thank goodness it did, for after that, the temptation drained from him. His rational, sober mind saw this as far too much for a single beer, not to mention the fact he would be throwing away all the progress he had already made. And so, the first day away from home came to a close, as they paid the bill and left the restaurant and headed back to the hotel, sober as a couple of Mormons.

Following that first night, where Andrew had looked Al square in the face and shunned him, he and Snhoj quickly developed a fitness routine. They would rise early and go for a run before breakfast, go and do a day's work and then go for a second run once they got back from work, before having a wash and going somewhere for dinner. They even went across the road to Argos, where they purchased some basic home gym equipment, which they set up in their hotel room for extra training. All the while, Al was far from his thoughts. He felt healthy, fit and on the road to recovery. If determination (and a sprinkling of stinginess) hadn't been on his side on that first evening in Horsham, the weeks could have gone by in a much different fashion, a whirlwind of intoxication and hangovers.

After the first two weeks, they travelled back up north for the weekend, to spend a few days at home, before travelling back down. They continued to do this every couple of weeks, never breaking from their fitness routine, continuing to behave when at home and when away.

They returned back to work after the second weekend spent at home. They continued their daily exercises throughout the week and were happy with the progress of the job. Friday of that week came around and Andrew and Snhoj were looking forward to a couple of days rest from work when the client who had got them the job appeared on the scene. She informed them that certain parts of the house needed to be completed that day, due to a party that was to take place there that weekend, so the pair ended up working late, not leaving the house until 9pm. They were tired and very hungry. The usual routine, naturally, went by the wayside that day, as there simply wasn't enough time if they were going to be able to go anywhere to eat. On their way back to the Travelodge, Andrew called the local Wagamama's, a place they had frequented many times whilst down in Horsham, so the staff had become familiar with them. "Will we be able to get in for something to eat shortly? We're just going back to the hotel for a wash and then we'll be straight there," Andrew asked.

"No problem, you'll probably just make it in time, see you both soon." So, they did exactly that. They rushed back, got sorted as quickly as possible and arrived just in time to eat. Whilst finishing up their food, the Wagamama's staff were planning to go for some drinks after their shift. After all, it was Friday night. Having become friendly with Andrew and Snhoj, some of the staff approached them and asked, "do you fancy joining us afterwards at Wabi's?" Wabi's, as it turned out, was a bar roughly 50 yards past the restaurant, which, under different circumstances, the pair would have probably sought out on the first night, but in their Al-shunning state, they hadn't even clocked. They agreed to go along with them. At this point, they weren't intending on drinking anything alcoholic, they just thought it might make a nice change to socialise a little after a long week of work.

Upon entering the bar, Andrew noticed a man drop a £5 note out of his back pocket while retrieving his wallet. He quickly stepped forward, picked up the note and tapped the shoulder of the man who had dropped it, proudly representing the friendly nature of us Northern lot. The man, who just so happened to be Paul Drayton, the partner (now husband) of TV Chatty Man, Alan Carr turned to Andrew. "Thank you so much, that's very kind of you!" he said, with genuine gratitude "Please, let me buy you two a drink to say thank you." Whether it was the long week of work, the crowded, lively bar, or the prospect of a free drink, it didn't take long for Andrew to respond.

"Aye go on then, be rude not to!" And just like that, what had eventually ended up as 9 weeks abstinence came to a grinding halt. The pint glass found the way to his hand, like an alcoholic-seeking missile and delivered its blow, 570ml of lager. And once that first layer had been peeled away in a flash, three more would come away over the course of the night. Four pints total. It was hardly what you would call binge drinking, but it was certainly enough for a man who had got it out of his system to feel awful the next day. However, it wasn't the hangover that was eating him the most; it was guilt. Buckets and buckets of guilt. 9 weeks of defying the naysayers, the people who told him he wouldn't manage to quit, the ones who told him he shouldn't quit since he "didn't have a problem to begin with." He proved them all wrong for 9 whole weeks, only to end it all so flippantly. But the worst part about it all, was that he felt like he'd let Christine down. She'd been so proud of him and had encouraged him every step of the way. She was thrilled to see him losing weight, exercising more, she enjoyed being able to converse with him of an evening, instead of watching him slur away with Al. Andrew knew full well how much this would upset and disappoint her, so he did what he thought would be best; he didn't tell her. He brushed the guilt under the proverbial carpet and pretended it didn't exist. When he spoke to her on the phone that morning, he tried his best to sound chipper and normal, like the enthusiastic, go-getter he had been for the past two and a bit months. And, unfortunately, Christine bought it.

Andrew and Snhoj returned back to work that morning, on the Saturday. The all too familiar aftereffects of a night on the drink were present, but they weren't enough to dampen their spirits. If anything, they actually sent Andrew hyper. He realised that he could enjoy a drink if he wanted too and not feel too dreadful the day after. Four pints a night is enough to enjoy himself, be feeling relatively okay the day after and continue to work unabated. In this daze of feeling invincible, he started to formulate plans: he was going to start and operate a cleaning business, alongside his decorating firm. And a plumbing firm. The world was his oyster, in his own, befuddled mind. And Snhoj had to listen to him indulge himself in his over-exhilarated state for the whole day. It was the sort of gibberish he spoke when spread out in the living room on a nightly basis, after four pints and a bottle of red, only now, this was coming from the mind of sober Andrew. A scary thought, if ever I've had one.

At the end of their shift, they did the usual and headed back to the hotel for a wash and then to head into town for something to eat, except, this time, they knew exactly what they were doing; they were going to drink, from the outset. All the defences Andrew had put up over 9 weeks, now removed by the previous night's four attacks, lay bent and broken by the wayside as they headed back to Wabi's to eat, drink and be merry, for tomorrow we regret. Any earlier feelings of guilt that had plagued Andrew had subsided and excitement took their place the closer he got to the pouring of the first drink. As much as he loves her, Christine was far from his mind, replaced by his old, faithful friend, Al, who had sat patiently over the past couple of months in anticipation of the wagon slowing to a stop.

In Andrew's words, they sat down to one of the best culinary experiences of their lives. Dish after dish was freshly prepared and brought to their table constantly throughout the night, the bill climbing ever higher. But, of course, the food was secondary to the drink. They sat and guzzled bottle after bottle of local, Sussex white wine at £27 a bottle. The Andrew that had rejected a £6 beer a few weeks ago was a far cry from the man who was now throwing this stuff down like it was tap water. More food, more drink, more food, more drink... like a constantly rotating conveyor belt of gluttony, the night rolled on, until the early hours of the morning, when Andrew could barely walk without assistance and his words made as much sense as Donald Trump's on the subject of global pandemics. They got a taxi back to the hotel and collapsed into their beds where they would awaken the next morning with heads as thick as steel beams.

They awoke at the usual time as they were supposed to be working that day, but when they came to their senses and realised the state they were in from the previous, debauched night, they called work off, using the excuse that Jordan's house would likely be a write off, due to the party last night. In reality, they could barely bring themselves to get out of bed, a rare thing for Andrew, a man who will deny hangovers until the cows come home and will try his best to act completely naturally. I suppose this can be traced back to his early drinking days, wanting to prove himself as a big drinker. Those "men" don't get hangovers, and neither should he! But this defiant attitude was all but defeated that morning as he lay there, stinking of booze and drowning in guilt.

As the day slowly ticked by, Andrew received a call from Christine, which he tried to play his best, "hello love, you alright?" he answered, as though all was fine.

"Hello, just checking in. How's work going?"

"Oh, we've not gone in today. Sacked it off. The house will be trashed from the party, so we've taken the day off." Andrew exclaimed. At this point, Christine still had no idea that Andrew had come off the wagon. As far as she was aware, he was heading into his tenth week of sobriety. But at this excuse, she started to sense that something was off.

"Oh, right. I thought you'd be cracking on so you could be done sooner and then you could come home. Have you called your Mum, by the way, to wish her Happy Birthday?" Of course, he hadn't. His conscious state was far too drowned to have remembered something like that.

"Oh bollocks, no, I forgot. I'll ring her now. Anyway, I best go. Going to go get some dinner. Thanks for ringing, love. Bye." And with that, he ended the conversation, with the elephant in the room hidden squarely under the carpet, along with all the grime and dirt from the night before.

For the majority of the rest of the day, the pair wallowed in self-pity, only getting out of bed to make frequent trips to the McDonalds across the road, simply to top up the food they'd already brought across, like a couple of students, blowing their student finance on take aways and partying. At some point in the day, Andrew had attempted a run, but had despised every second of it, feeling weak and unfit and with a constant lingering taste of booze lapping his tongue.

As the evening drew nearer on what had been a complete write off of a day, the pair grew giddy and excited; they had decided to do it all over again. The guilt pangs were starting to subside as the prospect of more booze drew nearer and nearer, until they were sat, once again, in Wabi's, repeating the exact same course of actions as the night before. The food kept coming, the Sussex wine kept disappearing down their necks. Deja vu. Over the course of the night, they had seen their Wagamama's friends dotted around the venue, which of course had prompted Andrew, life and soul of the party that he is, to loudly call them over and have a drink with them. They all stayed there until kicking out time, when their new friends suggested they go to a bar not far away who had karaoke on that night, where they could get more drink and Andrew could successfully make a complete arse of himself. Which he did. To perfection.

When sober, it would be wrong to describe Andrew as reserved, but if there is one social quality he upholds, it's respect. He keeps his voice down in restaurants, not wanting to disturb others, he makes sure not to swear in social situations and so on. He very well maintains a social standard. When he's been with Al, however, some of those standards tend to slip. By the time they arrived at the bar, they no longer existed. The Waga's staff took it in turns to perform some karaoke classics, pulling out hit after hit. Then it was Andrew's turn. He succinctly announced, "you Southern fucks have seen nothing yet! This Northern legend is going to blow you away!" at which he began belting out "Killing in the Name of" by Rage Against the Machine. Jumping around the bar like an escaped asylum patient, screeching the words "FUCK YOU, I WON'T DO WHAT YOU TELL ME!" repeatedly, the Waga's staff looked on him with sheer awe, many of them professing their love for him, agreeing with his proclamation that he was, indeed, a "legend" and asking Snhoj how they could possibly get a job doing anything to work alongside him.

It's worth noting that, as his son, I cringe an incomprehensible amount at the thought of these antics and I am eternally grateful to have not stood witness while he publicly humiliated himself in this way. What a bellend.

The next day, Monday, saw them finally return to work, where they were both incredibly hungover, but they were relishing in it, laughing about the night before and shrugging off any notion that they should probably stop. There was no way they were going to stop now. Especially not today, as another friend and decorator, Jason "Boo" Whalley, was currently making the journey down south to join them on the job. And to join them on their drinking escapades. After finishing work, with Boo now in tow, they headed to Wabi's for the third night in a row, under the guise of letting Boo experience the wonderful food on offer, but it was clear what the true intentions were, as wine and beer couldn't arrive at the table quick enough. Once again, they stayed until kicking out time, when the three of them then headed to the same bar as the previous night (Andrew, always a creature of habit). To their surprise, the bar was much quieter than the night before. Afterall, it was a Monday night. But that didn't stop them from continuing to party, drinking pint after pint. It was Boo's round and he returned from the bar with the beers, but also with the dreaded Jägerbombs, a new experience for Andrew. Once of a day, he would have steered clear of spirits and liqueurs and he is certainly not a fan of energy drinks, but lost in this destructive cosmos, he fired it down his neck without a second thought. After that, the night continued in this fashion. Each fresh drink came with another Jägerbomb chaser. Such an alarming cocktail of caffeinated energy drinks and strong alcohol is calamitous enough on a weekend of partying, but this was a Monday night. They had work the next day. The sane, sensible, on the wagon Andrew was completely dead and buried, replaced by a maniac, throwing caution to the wind, dancing on his grave and singing 90's rock anthems, with his arm around his best friend.

As the old saying goes, what goes up, must come down and unfortunately for Andrew, it was time to come down. Four straight nights of drinking after having been off the stuff for an extended period of time was bound to have some side effects, but there was no way Andrew could brace himself for what was about to happen to him. He woke up, still intoxicated and began getting ready for work. By now, the common morning guilt he had been suffering had reached boiling point and it started to gnaw away at his sanity. After showering and trying to bring himself back to his senses, he sat down and worked out how much he had spent in the last four days. The total astounded him - £600. It was unfathomable. Here sits a man who has mountainous money problems, has avoided drinking for 9 weeks, was starting to get his life back on track and within four days, he had ruined it all. And for what gain? He was ill, he was skint, he had lied to Christine by not telling her... He had absolutely nothing to show for the past four nights except an unstable mental condition, which he tried to subdue, tried to see past as he continued to get ready for work alongside Snhoj and Boo. But he couldn't hide from it for long. As the three of them arrived at the McDonalds across the road for some breakfast, Andrew stayed outside, barely even conscious of where he currently was, so lost in a self-inflicted daze. He wanted to ring Christine and confess to his actions, but he couldn't bring himself to do it, but in desperation to open himself up to somebody, other than the people who had been on a bender alongside him, he called his old friend Jeff. "Hello, Buddy, how are you doing my mate?" Jeff answered.

"Hello Jeff, I'm alright, are..." But Andrew couldn't finish his sentence. He burst into uncontrollable tears, sat on a cold bench outside a roadside McDonalds in Horsham. Everything had finally caught up with him and the pressure had grown too much. He began to feel as though he could never escape Al. All the effort he had put in recently had just led him here, right back to where he had started. In fact, not where he had started, but even lower than that. The past few nights made his daily basket look like a warm up. He was scared. Scared that he had done irreparable damage. And he still had to tell his wife, who had been so proud of all he had achieved. After struggling to express his bountiful guilt to Jeff and with him unable to make any sense of the situation, the phone call came to an end, and Andrew straight away called Christine and told her everything, still whilst frantically crying. She was stunned. She had sensed something was afoot when they had last spoken, but she hadn't realised to what extent that something was. Coming off the wagon and going back to his old ways was one thing, but plummeting off and spending such a ridiculous amount was shocking. Confessing didn't have the effect Andrew had hoped it would. Nothing was alleviated, he just continued to feel worthless.

Boo and Snhoj saw Andrew outside and came out to see what had happened, but they could barely get anything coherent out of him, so they took him back across to the hotel and went to work without him, leaving him to rest and, hopefully, recover. But he didn't. Instead, when Boo returned to the hotel during his lunch break, he found Andrew pacing back and forth in his room, still crying, still struggling to formulate sentences through his tortured state. He was having a full-blown breakdown, and Boo and Snhoj didn't know how to handle the situation. To see the "legend" in a state such as this, inconsolable as he was, scared them. After Boo returned back to work, Andrew tried to compose himself and decided to go and get some air by wandering around Horsham. But once he was outside, he found he couldn't concentrate on anything. He would occasionally come to his senses and realise he had been stood in a daze, staring into space. He rang Christine numerous times, who had by this point spoken to the doctors to try and get any advice to help a man suffering an alcohol induced nervous breakdown, hundreds of miles away. But no advice she imparted on him helped. He just continued to blindly wander the streets.

Once things had calmed down somewhat, the three of them developed a new routine of staying in after work, eating takeaways and drinking cans of lager. Of course, this wasn't ideal, but it was better than continuing on with the rampage. Andrew returned home the following weekend, where he did no exercise or anything to try to remedy the damage, he just had a couple of baskets before returning down south, this time with just Boo, to finish the job. They stayed down there for another few weeks, where they would drink four or five pints nightly and do no exercise at all. It was just like the good old days of Andrew's addiction.

And with that, the first wheel had come off Andrew's 3-wheel wagon. He had made a valiant effort to kick the habit, only for things to escalate to levels unimagined. The weeks following the completion of the Horsham job were some of the most trying of Andrew and Christine's lives, in terms of their relationship. They would argue almost daily about the fact he was back in his old ways, was spending money like we had an endless supply of it and that he was doing nothing to prevent himself from having another breakdown. The thought of him attempting to try to quit again became scary, because if the inevitable relapse was going to be anything like the one he had just experienced, what would the damage be like this time? But that would be defeatist. He had to try again. He had to get back on his wagon, before it was too late.

Chapter 9

Two Wheels on my Wagon

When you have an all or nothing attitude, it can be very difficult to stick to your guns. I have absolutely inherited that attribute from my Dad and it can be quite infuriating at times. For example: I decided I was going to join a gym. Now, anyone developing an exercise regime would probably best advise you to slowly ease into regular exercise, maybe doing one or two, possibly three sessions a week, just while you find your footing and get used to this new way of life. But someone with an all or nothing attitude, like me and my Dad, would straight away go to the gym every day. It's all we would think about. We'd check our weight every day, hoping to see the changes, we'd discuss the gym with everyone we talked to, we'd be doing sit ups and push-ups at home and just generally be consumed by the thought of exercise. And eventually, you'd become worn out from over-exercise. Then you might miss a day at the gym. And then your new routine is off-kilter, and so you may as well scrap the whole thing. Now, maybe if I'd eased into a new exercise routine and not made myself live and breathe exercise, I would have found it easier to work into my weekly schedule and would have been able to stick it out longer, but it is not in my nature to do that.

Let's now apply that to my Dad's addiction. Whenever he has made an attempt to stop drinking, as I've already stated, it's been a full stop, underlined decision to quit. Maybe he would have found it easier to wean himself off the drink? Cutting down his daily intake of alcohol slowly over the course of a couple of weeks, until he is less reliant on it and then can stop altogether, almost without even realising he has done it. Unfortunately, though, he can't allow himself to do that. Because if he is having one can of lager, he is on the drink, so why not have four? And a bottle of red? This is just the way his brain is wired, so there is no avoiding this logic for him. So, in the event that he has a period of no drink, but really fancies having a cold beer one day, it can't just be that one beer, unfortunately. Perhaps this is the ultimate source of his addictive personality? I know that, ideally, he would love to be able to have the occasional drink, like most "normal" people can, as he sees it. But he knows in himself that that can't happen, and so he *has* to quit altogether, or not at all.

· · · · · · · · · · ·

June 2013 - Almost exactly two years after the last big effort to get on the wagon, and many more smaller, aborted attempts to try again, it was time for Andrew's next big attempt at kicking the habit. Since his previous relapse, he had gone back to his regular evenings of relying on the basket. Nothing had changed as a result of the experience except that he now knew that he could stop for a period of time and that maybe if he tried again, it could maybe last even longer than the previous time.

He decided that, this time, he was going to get some help. Maybe he couldn't do it on his own? Of course, he always had Christine by his side, helping where she could, but perhaps the help of a professional was what he needed? So, he began to seek it out. Andrew got in touch with his uncle, who is someone who has struggled with addiction for many years. At the time of contacting him, however, he had been sober for a long time. Andrew asked him how he managed to stop drinking, which prompted his uncle to invite him along to an Alcoholics Anonymous meeting, which he had been attending regularly and had helped him to quit. I remember being very proud of Andrew and thinking that it was incredible for him to admit his problem and to try new methods of getting help.

However, after a couple of sessions, he decided that it wasn't working for him. This isn't to say AA doesn't work and wouldn't work for somebody else. Over the course of writing this book, I have spoken to people who have found real success with AA and the programme it provides, and are living proof that it can work for some people, but for Andrew and his impatient, wandering mind, it wasn't working out. Still, he had taken the first step and had reached out for help, and it certainly wasn't the only option available.

Next he tried going to the doctors, to see what they could advise. They solidified his status as an alcoholic, whereas before he'd questioned it, as he wasn't the stereotype of an alcoholic; someone who wakes up with a vodka bottle in hand, stinking of booze and commences drinking in the morning. He wasn't convinced the label applied to him. He just identified that he had a problem saying no to a nightly drink. The doctor confirmed that that was indeed the symptoms of an alcoholic. He informed Andrew and Christine (who had gone along with him to ensure that Andrew would follow up on the advice imparted on him) that if a person only drinks one drink a day, but is reliant on that one drink, then they are indeed an alcoholic (which, I must admit, makes me more than a little concerned about my reliance on caffeine). So now he had a better grasp of the concept of alcoholism and knew that the label did apply to himself. The doctor prescribed him some form of tablets - of which Andrew can't remember the name - that were intended to quell the craving for alcohol. Unfortunately, as with the AA meetings, this method also failed for Andrew. The issue was clearly too deep-rooted. But again, the exercise wasn't completely futile, as he now had a wider knowledge of his own condition.

After a few more failed efforts to seek help, such as visiting wellness centres, speaking to more former addicts and even attending hypnotherapy sessions, Andrew decided, once again, to take the problem into his own hands. He'd done so well the last time, what's to say he couldn't do it again this time, but better, equipped with the experience of the previous effort and an expanded knowledge of the subject.

At the time, Andrew was working at a large stately home not far from Barnoldswick. The job was huge and provided a constant flow of work. It paid well and on time, so money was starting to roll in on a regular basis, which was exciting for him. His decision to quit couldn't have come at a better time in this regard, as he started to see what it was like to have money accumulate in his bank account, rather than it depleting as quickly as it arrived. A few weeks of living this way was highlighting benefits left, right and centre. As before, he felt more fit and active. His bike rides were easier, his gym sessions didn't leave him as breathless, his anxieties were minimised. All was going swimmingly. He was working alongside a young decorator called Sam, who was, coincidentally, my friend and the singer in the band I was in at the time. Andrew and Sam grew closer and closer as they worked together, day in day out. They began to formulate the idea of a holiday to Majorca. Andrew, Sam, Christine, Sam's partner, Sally and my best friend Andy would all go away together for a week, which was an incredibly tantalizing idea. We were all hugely excited about the prospect and so we booked it as soon as possible. But, of course, Al was lurking in the corner of Andrew's mind. This would be the ultimate test of his determination to not drink. Foreign holidays in the past had meant one thing for Andrew - booze. Nothing accompanied incredible, local, Spanish cuisine like wine. Nothing tasted better than a brandy, sat looking at the harbour. Nothing was more refreshing than a cold beer, sitting in the sun outside a local, colourful cafe. In his mind, it was idyllic conditions for drinking. He knew this was going to be a challenge, but in the run up to the holiday, he remained defiant in his reluctance to not drink, sure that he could get through a week of sun without it.

When he would discuss the upcoming break with people, he would proudly announce that it would be his first holiday abroad without drinking since he turned 18. They would scoff at him, calling him mad for even attempting it. Some would even exclaim, "why? That's what a holiday is all about!" But Andrew was unperturbed by their pessimistic attitude. He had his own plans for the holiday. He was going to hire a road bike for the time we were there, so he could go on beautiful coastal rides, a new, fresh, exciting experience, that he was excited to have replace his old habits.

The day finally arrived. Myself, Andy, Sam and Sally had all slept in our living room, excitedly discussing how much we were looking forward to the holiday. We made it to the airport after a disastrous minibus journey, rife with traffic jams and an old engine that struggled up the hills towards Leeds Bradford airport. But despite these troubles, we made it in enough time and got sat in a cafe in the airport lounge to have some breakfast. Sam, in the spirit of the holiday, was keen to order himself a pint of lager, but was trepidatious to do so, not wanting to appear to be rubbing it in Andrew's face. But Andrew was fine with it, telling Sam to go ahead and enjoy himself. Just because he wasn't drinking, that should be in no way detrimental to the plans of the rest of us - it was our holiday too, after all. So, Sam got his beer, and all was well. He had another couple on the flight, which Andrew continued to pass off as no issue. Inside, however, the battle had already begun. There was nothing he would have liked more than to join Sam in seeing the holiday in in this way, but he stuck to his guns, drinking lime and soda and looking forward to his bike riding adventures.

We arrived at the villa in the beautiful town of Port de Pollença, all buzzing with excitement for the week ahead. Andrew went to pick his hire bike up from the rental shop and things were looking good. But then came the first night. We headed out on to the seafront to decide where we would be eating that night. As we gleefully walked along, Andrew's silent internal battle with himself continued onwards, as he noticed every sip taken by every person sat outside the various restaurants and bars situated along the way. To him, it was like a real-life version of the Jim Carrey film, The Truman Show. It was as though everybody had an earpiece in, awaiting their direction. "Okay, he's rounding the corner to come past the bar now. Take a sip of your beer in 5, 4, 3..." and sure enough, as Andrew came into view, the patrons of the establishments would take long, joyful gulps of their alcoholic beverages and it drove Andrew insane. Perhaps Al had coordinated the whole thing, monitoring

Andrew's moves from the lighthouse, not far out at sea. But, through sheer will and determination, Andrew resisted these cruel mind games. The first meal went down without the aid of the forbidden fluid and Andrew went to bed that night sober as a stone. A first, while in a foreign climate.

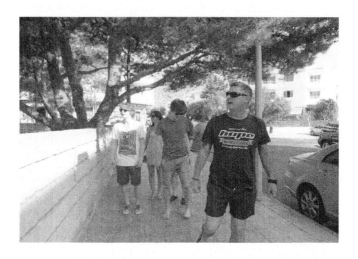

The next day, he arose before the rest of us, got on his lycra and went for his first bike ride of the holiday, riding out towards Al's lair, the lighthouse. He circled around it, symbolically giving Al the middle finger and riding back before coming to meet the rest of us at the local swimming pool. Despite perspiring like a snowman on a sunbed, he felt incredible. Exercise over alcohol, on a holiday abroad. What an achievement! But the second evening meal of the holiday proved a challenge, once again. We discovered a small, quiet seafood restaurant down a side street. Once we got seated, Sam asked if Andrew would mind if he had a beer. Again, Andrew reminded him that this was his holiday too and that if he wanted a beer, he should have a beer. And so he did. The waiter brought it over and placed it in front of Sam, who was sitting on the opposite side of the table from Andrew. It had been a particularly hot day and Andrew had worked out hard and as he sat there, staring at the golden liquid in front of him, the condensation dripping down the side of the chalice, the bubbles rising from the activator at the bottom of the glass, there was nothing he wanted more than to pick it up and let it flow slowly down his throat. It took every ounce of his determination to not do so and he miraculously resisted for a second night running.

Day 3. We decided that we would all hire bikes for the day to join Andrew on a ride into Old Town Pollenca, a place Andrew and Christine (along with myself and Chris, at younger ages) had stayed many times. The ride was hot, sweaty and tiring, but we eventually arrived in the picturesque square of the Old Town, where sat the couple's favourite restaurant. We approached to see that the owner, Martin, who they had grown to know over their numerous visits on previous holidays, was setting up tables outside. He greeted Andrew and Christine with big, friendly hugs and encouraged us to get booked in for a meal that night. With little persuasion necessary, we did so, before riding back to the Port to wash and get ready for the night ahead. Andrew knew that this evening would be the ultimate challenge of the holiday. On their previous holiday there, they had discovered that Martin made what they would argue was the best mojito in the world. Even Christine, who rarely drinks to excess, had become enamoured with them and couldn't wait to have one that very evening. Andrew knew that he would struggle to resist such temptation. And struggle he did. As we ordered our food and drinks, Christine pulled the trigger and ordered the first mojito of the evening. Martin personally brought it to her, and she took her first sip, reaffirming it as one of the tastiest things she had ever drunk. Beads of sweat started to pour down Andrew's forehead as the assault took place. What felt like a lifetime of deliberation battled in Andrew's mind within 30 seconds, when he finally opened his mouth to exclaim, "well, I can't not have one, we're not here every day. I'll have one as well please, Martin." And so it was done, the bullet was loaded into the chamber. But it was only intended to be fired once. However, as soon as the rum in the mojito touched Andrew's lips, it was over. The wagon known as sobriety came skidding to a halt for the second time, losing its second wheel. After that, the holiday continued in the traditional way. Beer, wine, cocktails, brandys... Al looked on from his lighthouse. His job here was done.

Thankfully, the shock of the situation didn't hit as hard as the previous relapse. Afterall, nothing was being kept secret from us and, in a way, we didn't really blame him for what he did. Even Christine, who had been so massively heartbroken at his previous failed attempt to quit, had agreed that he couldn't not have a mojito in Martin's restaurant. But little did we know, at the time, that that would be Andrew's last attempt for a long time. He had admitted defeat and settled back into life as a drinker. We returned back to the UK after the week, where we saw Andrew resume his basket loving business as though he'd never been away from it, sat in his seat, Al by his side. He would remain that way for a long time. He continued to exercise, still enjoying his bike rides and gym sessions, but he couldn't escape the fact that he was trying to out-train a bad diet, living on his daily mix of booze, nuts and sweets, trying to justify things to himself with the exercise he did. A few years later, a storm blew in from the east.

Chapter 10

Oblivion: My Ultimate White-Knuckle Ride

The third and final wheel of this proverbial wagon came bundled with a certain beast, visiting from the east. By this point, my Dad had tried twice to climb onto the wagon and both times, a wheel had come loose and the apple cart had toppled. But what if he had the ability to get back on it, even with just the one wheel remaining? In that sense, this story would chronicle the third and final wheel of that wagon and as you know, with the beast taming that occurred back at the start of this journey, that wheel has carried him a long, long way. Far removed from the man who successfully broke two wheels through excessiveness. A man who had told the world time and time again that it was over, only to run back to his basket on a nightly basis. One whose fear had kept him snared in that beer-scented trap, who longed to be free, but could not break the shackles and live the life he sought for himself. To do that, he would have to overcome that fear. His ultimate white-knuckle ride had been waiting for him all his life and before it could gather too much rust, it was time to take his seat.

．．．．．．．．．．．

As Andrew spent each day consuming Craig Beck's book, the fear of the unknown consumed him. Life events were all about drinking, so what would they be like without it? What did Christmas look like without a can of Stella being opened before 11am? What even was a meal out without a bottle of red all to himself? Is a holiday without drink even a holiday? It was hard to imagine any of these things without an alcoholic sheen cast over them. Like a cavernous pit with no light, a sober life was an uncharted and incredibly daunting prospect. But the knowledge being delivered into his ears was also exciting. Think about when you did something you knew you shouldn't as a child. That thrill of maybe getting caught and told off by an adult, as you climbed into the construction zone with your friends. Your heart beating rapidly with adrenaline, looking round each corner to make sure nobody was coming before running from building to building. Andrew felt that thrill as Craig delivered secret after secret into his cranium. He was learning how to defy Al and although that was an incredibly positive thing for him to do, it was massively against the grain that was his everyday life and so it felt as though he was tearing up his own rulebook more and more with each passage devoured. But unlike those carefree, childhood experiences, this came packaged with the undeniable truth that this *had* to be done. There was no chickening out like in the past. This *had* to be the point of no return. But what if it didn't work? What if he spent all his time following the steps laid out for him, only for him to slip, break the wheel and come tumbling back down to earth? It could all go wrong in the blink of an eye, just like that rollercoaster.

Before the crushing news of his van repossession had been imparted on him, Andrew and his work crew had had an unforgettable day at Alton Towers. They had arrived bright and early in the morning, before the queues had started to grow to ridiculous lengths. The weather was glorious, and the laughs had started the minute they piled into the van and started the journey. Everything had seemed perfect. Like giddy boys, they excitedly discussed which ride they would head to first. Should they start with the big ones, before more people arrive? Or should they start small and build up to the big ones? Whatever they decided upon, there was one thing certain in Andrew's mind, Oblivion sounded horrendous. A ride which features a sheer vertical drop into a cavernous hole, one which is veiled behind a wall of mist. After a painfully slow, sharp incline, taking you up to the drop zone, the cart slowly carries you round and holds you temporarily over the unknown pit below, before it lets go of the breaks and plunges you down. To Andrew, a man with no stomach for the scary things in life, the idea of going on this ride was hideous. As they stood around the viewing platform that gives you the perfect view of the cart as it plunges, the screams of the ride's victims sent more fear shooting down Andrew's spine. No way. It's not going to happen. Not yet at least.

The day continued, with the crew working their way through all the biggest and best rides on offer. Andrew had conquered them all (nearly backing out of some of the more intimidating ones at the last minute), but his biggest foe still stood undefeated in the dreaded "X-Sector" of the park. Oblivion. They made their way back to the corner of the park where the beast continued to swallow its prey, deep into its foreboding chasm. After watching a few more carriages plummet into the unknown, and with a healthy amount of peer pressure being shoveled on to him, Andrew decided it was time to face his fears and take the plunge. Literally. Palms sweating, he joined the queue. As the rest of the gang were laughing and joking about Boo's face paint, Andrew was quietly regretting his decision, and wondering if he could sneak out without anybody noticing. But it was too late. He'd made the commitment and told them all he was doing it. If he backs out now, the grief from his friends will be endless. Eventually, they made it to the front and took their seats in the long rows that make up the carriages of Oblivion. The restraints came down, the belts were in place and the young man working the controls had his thumb on the launch button. Final checks were made, and the carriage rolled out of the station. By now, Andrew was the shade of snow. His stomach was rolling over at a rate he couldn't keep up with and his mouth was verbalising the fear dwelling within him through various colourful language choices. The carriage crawled to the top of the lift chain and began to round the corner, lining up with that oh so terrifying descent. Just as it always does, moments before the vertical drop, the ride stopped and held for a brief pause. But in that moment, we see Andrew reflected in this screaming analogy. His future decisions and life are plastered all over this moment in time, where he sits on a ride he swore he wouldn't go near, facing his fears, the unknown feeling of what will happen once the brakes release and the carriage is enveloped in the shroud of mist below. What awaits on the other side? How will it feel, to take the plunge? What will people say when it's over? Will I be happier for having done this? Why did I even bother in the first place? This is bloody stupid!

When Andrew first made that decision on February 27th, 2018, he had no idea what journey awaited him, or of the changes that would become apparent over time. Of course, he knew that he would be healthier and that he would have more money as a result of the decision, but since the age of 18, when he first threw back that rum, he didn't know what a sober life felt like. I could tell you again about the Christmases, the parties, the holidays, but in reality, it was every day. Alcohol was as important to his daily functions as his lungs and his heart, so how should he know what it feels like to strip it away? And then there were the doubters. The ones who told him that they'd heard it all before and laughed it off as another thing that Andrew Dickin was gonna do. That scared him even more. He doubted himself, due to these naysayers (of which I admit to being one). "They're right," he thought to himself. "I have said this all before. Why will this time be any different?" But having to explain to people that this time it *will* be different was exhausting and just multiplied the pressure that was being piled upon him, not least from himself. "People are going to call me boring!" But, so what, at least I'll have money. "People aren't going to want to invite me to things anymore because I'm not drinking!" How do you know? They've never met sober Andrew. "But what about when I go for a meal with Christine? She loves to have a drop of wine then!" No,

Andrew, she doesn't. That's how you legitimised drinking in your own head. With each new fear passing before his mind, he would push rewind on the Craig Beck audiobook and listen back to the most recent secret delivered, each one feeling like a new weapon being added to the arsenal.

When the book came to an end and Andrew had poured over every detail within, learning to accept and face his fears, he felt like he had opened up a box containing the best kept secret. The rulebook to a fresh, new, clean and sober life. The game changer to end all game changers.

The brakes released, and the carriage plunged.

Chapter 11

Grays Sports Almanac

Marty McFly came from a fairly below average American background. Granted, he was still in high school, but he couldn't afford his own car, his Dad was a victim of workplace bullying, his Mum was an alcoholic, his uncle had earned the nickname "Jailbird" Joey, due to the amount of times he'd been in and out of prison... All round, the McFly/Baines family had things pretty rough. I'm sure if Marty had a way of predicting the future, in order to manipulate the outcome, hence making life better for himself and his family, he would do precisely that. So, when Emmett "Doc" Brown crashed his way onto the driveway of the McFly household, knocking over their bins and announcing that Marty and his girlfriend Jennifer had to accompany him to the future, a window of opportunity presented itself to Marty in the form of a sporting events results almanac. Found in an antique goods shop in the year 2015 (bearing in mind young Mr McFly had arrived here from the year 1985), Grays Sports Almanac was a complete record of sporting events results from the year 1950 right up to 2000. It didn't take long for Marty to realise that if he was to purchase this book, he could take it back with him to 1985 and become exceedingly wealthy by betting on sports events, knowing that he would pick the winner every time. He could finally get that pickup truck he'd always wanted and show Needles, who was boss in a drag race (just look out for Rolls Royce's). He makes the purchase, only for Doc to happen upon the book and discover what Marty had planned. He accosted Marty for being so reckless, informing him that he did not invent the time machine for financial gain, and that doing something as reckless as this could lead to detrimental results. The future was best left unwritten. Now, anyone who has seen Back to The Future Part 2 will know exactly what happened to said almanac after it fell into the hands of that bastard Biff, but what if Doc had been wrong? Who was he to say that had Marty taken the almanac home with him to 1985 and put it to good use, things wouldn't have been all round better for the McFly's? That timeline is something we can only imagine, but that's not to say that certain other books couldn't provide similar results. And better yet, what if this could happen for real, and not just on the silver screen?

May I present to you, Andrew's Alcoholics Almanac:

. . . .

"I no longer have to speak to the bitter, overweight, twisted piece of shit anymore" - Andrew Dickin, on himself

Andrew doesn't regret the fact that drink played a role in his life. During the times we have had discussions about this book, we have laughed a lot about some of the stories that have come about as a result of him drinking (some of which I can't really share here, but please, take my word for it) and some of his happiest/fondest memories have been during drinking sessions with friends and family. That's not to say that he couldn't have enjoyed these moments had drink not been involved, but I certainly believe it is an unhealthy way to live regretting the past and wondering what might have been. It's also worth noting that had Andrew not been a drinker from a young age and therefore hadn't been in the pub the night Christine plucked up the courage to pinch his arse as he walked past, pint in hand, they may never have started their relationship. I might not be sitting here typing this story about how my father was a drinker. In fact, I wouldn't be here at all. What a paradox. But I digress; drinking has been a big part of his life, for better or for worse. But, if perhaps Andrew could have seen the results of a life without drink back when he was, say, 30 years old, maybe he would have thrown the towel in there. Let's say that Andrew was sat watching TV one day, pouring his third can of Stella into his pint glass, when all of a sudden, a vision of himself from the future appeared on the screen. He's a lot slimmer, he's less blotchy and he appears much less anxious, but it's definitely him. He holds in his hand a copy of "My Basketful of Happiness", the number one bestseller about one man's struggle with addiction. He turns to this very page and begins reading aloud to Andrew the benefits of life when alcohol isn't involved:

No more high blood pressure - When Andrew had seen his old friend that day whilst out for a walk and she informed him she had suffered a stroke due to high blood pressure; he had begun to take this subject a little more seriously. The thought that he himself could soon suffer a stroke due to this very issue was terrifying, but it was also highly likely. His blood pressure was sky high due to the incredible pressure on his organs from over drinking and combatting that with intense exercise. If a stroke didn't strike him down, he risked going on to blood pressure medication for the rest of his life, another not-so-appealing prospect. But now, numerous years and no booze later, Andrew's blood pressure is perfectly average for his age and weight.

He can now exercise in peace, without worrying that the next rotation of the pedals could be his last.

Weight loss - I'm sure it will come as no great revelation to you, dear reader, that drinking is a surefire way to gain weight. There's a reason people can identify a "beer belly." But perhaps you may not realise the extent of the change that can be made simply by removing alcohol from your daily diet. Andrew has lost over 3 stone in weight since that fateful day in 2018 and that weight loss is owed entirely to the removal of alcohol from the equation. He hasn't changed his diet (apart from perhaps fewer takeaways as a side result of not being intoxicated) and his exercise routine is roughly the same as ever, except now, his daily functions aren't in a constant back and forth battle with Al and his 10 Steps to Weight Gain programme. It really is remarkable to look at side by side pictures of Andrew and to see the difference for yourself. Multiple chins have simply vanished since booze was removed from the equation. He'd gained a lot of weight over the years, and it wasn't until you compared the photos that that was so clear. He was happy taking the mick out of himself for it, along with everybody else, but secretly, he knew it wasn't a good thing, and despite laughing hysterically when somebody called him "Jabba" or compared him to something you might find in a zoo, he longed to be the slim, athletic man he once was.

No more money worries - After a lifetime of just scraping by, living on the bread line, squeezing every penny in the lead up to pay day, Andrew and Christine no longer have to worry about not making ends meet. For the first time in their married life, they have money in the bank. If they want to go away on holiday, they no longer need to sell family heirlooms to do so. They no longer have to borrow money from their children just to do the weekly food shop. They're no longer driving vehicles that could break down at any moment. The advantages of a life with financial stability are innumerable. Having been the number one driving force behind the decision to kick the habit, this newfound appreciation for money in the bank has been truly eye opening for the couple. The residual effects of the dark days, when losing the house was a real prospect, still linger to this day, as mentioned, but when the realisation settles in that the van on the street is simply delivering an Amazon package, they remember that they no longer owe money to anybody; there is no fear that the next vehicle on the cul-de-sac could be leaving with our living room contents loaded in the back. And, once again, this alleviation of money worries can be accredited to one simple thing; Andrew doesn't hang out with Al anymore.

He had made himself a promise, before he had given up. In usual Dickin fashion, Andrew had never owned a firsthand bike, other than when he was a child. It was the same with cars, besides maybe one or two new vehicles while Andrew had been in the motor trade. Televisions, exercise equipment, whatever it was that was being purchased, more often than not, they were pre-loved, simply because it was cheaper. But when the prospect of quitting first presented itself, Andrew had promised himself that with the money he would usually blow on the basket, he would buy himself a brand-new mountain bike. But, again, true to Andrew's traits, he wanted it straight away. Despite this growing list of benefits, he still remains an incredibly impatient man, so he decided he would take out a loan, in order to buy the bike straight away. In a sense, this became insurance. In order to meet the loan repayments, he would need to keep off the drink, or he couldn't afford to pay them. He had inadvertently caught himself in another Catch 22 situation, and it worked out beautifully. With the money saved, he met every payment and still had enough money flowing in to sort out a better family motor and take more than one drink-free holiday to the beautiful North East coast. It's an expensive hobby, that there drinking.

No more negativity - Andrew has lost friends through the years due to his negativity and his occasional anti-everything attitude. When he'd had a "skinful" the night before and he was suffering the consequences the day after, Andrew would prattle on about so and so is a knob head, this and that is a load of shit... Generally speaking, he was pretty angry and altogether not very pleasant to be around when in this state. Really, all it boiled down to was the fact that he had to be at work, where he couldn't drink beer and lounge around his living room, so his frustrations would be vented on just about anything and anyone who had a different view to his own. Of course, that all changed when he *was* lounging around in his living room and the beer was flowing. As you know by now, Andrew was on top of the world during these times and all was well with the world. Now, however, with a clear, uninhibited mind, Andrew doesn't live his life this way. It's been a miraculous thing to witness the change in him, to see him be so much more accepting of everyone and everything. He smiles more, he laughs more, and he is an all-round nicer, more generous person. He has repaired bridges that he had burnt, during bitter phases, reconnecting with people he thought he never would, and I can see just how much it means to him to be able to do that. Some of said people may be shocked to find Andrew as a sober, "normal" person now, surprised that they aren't reconnecting under the influence, but it is also clear to see the respect and admiration people have for him when they see the change for themselves in his appearance, personality and all-round spirit.

Speaking of spirit, Andrew discovered a morsel of faith, after giving up the booze. No, he didn't become born again, and he certainly doesn't wake up each morning and start praying to his God, rather his faith comes in the form of respect and acceptance. Whilst on a short weekend break with Christine (which, again, he can easily afford to do now without having to bankrupt himself in the process), Andrew had a chance encounter with a Unitarian chapel. The patrons of said establishments are essentially free to express their own search and meaning for truth and for quality of life. They are accepting of all faiths and beliefs, allowing everybody who attends a chance to express themselves, be it through their belief in their God, or through a life-changing experience. After his first day in the chapel, Andrew, along with Christine, started attending services every Sunday at Kendal Unitarian Chapel. He found this to be an incredibly positive experience, one that left him feeling gratified and even more accepting than before, each time he attended. He has even volunteered to do readings in the chapel. Hard to imagine him doing something like that after a night with the basket.

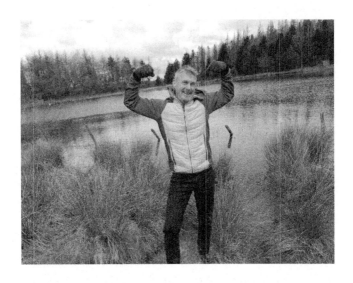

Lust for life - They say, "health is wealth." Well, it would appear that is true. Since ending his drinking career, Andrew has an entirely new lust for living. He sets his alarm clock every day for 5am the following morning, simply so he can get up and start making the most of the day. By 5.30am, he has already had a coffee and is sat listening to music in the sun lounge, making the most of not only being alive, but feeling fresh. No hangovers to contend with, no bitterness or anger to dwell on, no money-induced anxiety to fill him with dread. In a sense, giving up drinking has been his true enlightenment to how good his life can be without it. He actually feels sad on a Sunday evening now. Not because he doesn't enjoy his job, he truly does, but because weekends have taken on a new form. No longer are the day times just a nuisance in the way of his basket, they're a chance for him to enjoy himself, whether that be with the remedial tasks such as gardening or tidying, or with going out for bike rides, going to the gym or visiting friends and family. Andrew derives true happiness from these moments now, and it's that happiness and enjoyment that delivers the sadness when it comes to a close each week.

One particular story sticks in his mind, from a previous (failed) attempt to get on the wagon. He was on a trip to Wales with a group of cyclists for a weekend of riding. After a few miles of cycling, the group of over 10 stopped in the middle of a forest to have a quick break and plan their evening, after the ride. Naturally, the plan was to go to a pub and sample the local ale. With Andrew briefly being on the wagon at this point, he was thinking of his own plans in his head, when one of the members of the group stated the following: "what must it be like to be one of these non-drinkers who, when they wake up, that is the best they will feel all day." The group all chuckled and agreed that that was absolute madness. But it struck a chord with Andrew, because he realised that that was exactly what he wanted. He didn't want to have to spend money on becoming intoxicated in order to make himself feel better than he does when he first wakes up in the morning. He realises with hindsight that that quote comes from a mind that was similar to his own of the past, one that didn't know what it was like when the brakes release and the train emerges on the other side of the hole, to know that life is drastically different without those aids. It wasn't until he experienced waking up feeling "as good as he would feel all day" that he realised what an ignorant quote that was. PS: When they went to the pub that night, Andrew went and watched Superman at the cinema on his own.

Improved relationships - Speaking on a personal level, I can connect with my father a lot easier, now. I don't see and rarely speak to him during the day, with us both being at work, so coming home in the evening during his drinking days to find that he's already intoxicated, I decided there was no point in trying to start a conversation, because the responses will be nonsensical and he won't remember what we even discussed, so I'd just take myself off to my room or go and see my friends, keeping out of the way. Now, however, I can actually have somewhat intelligent conversations with him. We will discuss and listen to music, watch documentaries together and, of course, have meetings for this very book, something that, subject matter removed, we could have never done a few years ago.

Of course, as I already mentioned, he can also reconnect with people he'd been bitter towards in the past, as well as developing friendships and relationships with people who he wouldn't have given the time of day when he was bitter.

But one relationship in particular has seen the greatest improvement as a result of his quitting and stands above and beyond all other benefits that have come before this: his relationship with his wife, Christine. A woman who stood beside him during his worst times, when she would spend the evenings largely in silence, knowing that he was basking in Al's presence, re-watching Auf Wiedersehen Pet, mouthing off and guzzling. The day times and weekends would often lead to arguments, spurred on by hungover Andrew's bitterness and anger. Through devastating money woes, depression, breakdowns and all the dark days that came as a result of his addiction, Christine never abandoned him and for that, she deserves a medal of biblical proportions. And with Andrew's now clear vision, he is eternally grateful and amazed that she managed to withstand it all. He sees that past version of himself as a separate entity, and he knows that to live alongside that must have been an incredible challenge for all, but especially his wife. With that respect for such an achievement, the couple have grown closer than ever. Of course, they always loved each other, even through it all, but they connect in so many more ways now that they can share more between them. Andrew's' ex-favourite hobby was one Christine didn't want to join him in, but with his new and improved outlook on life, they do so much more together, even down to the little things such as watching TV shows together of an evening. That might seem trivial, but for a man who couldn't concentrate on a half hour show, unless it was something he'd seen a thousand times before, it's a huge change, and one that has made the evenings so much more pleasurable for Christine and the rest of us. And that pleasure is reflected in all facets of their relationship. The bond between them is now unbreakable, having weathered through so much.

The benefits Andrew has experienced could serve as a sequel to this book. He really is Andrew 2.0 since making the change. Leaving aside the key benefits mentioned above, Andrew **gave up antidepressants** after 7 years of taking them alongside drinking, creating a battle between the booze bringing him down and the pills bringing him up. It's no wonder his mood was so unbalanced most of the time. He had **sores on his legs**, which were refusing to dissipate, even with medication from the doctors. They appeared to be fungal infections, with the cause being bad circulation, due to the alcohol. After a year of not drinking, the sores had completely healed up, with no extra medication. He now **spends less time in the gym** but feels the benefits as though he was working out twice as hard for twice as long. This is because he is no longer trying to out-train a bad diet. He no longer rewards a workout session with an evening of binging, believing he deserved such reward, but really undoing all good accomplished. **No more anxiety, no more desperation, no longer lazy:** home decorated, cars cleaned, dogs walked and exercised… The list continues on and on and is only growing the more time he spends as a sober man.

In the previous chapter, I talked about how much fear Andrew felt, as he sat there on that first morning and made a note in his diary. The new beginning was now, but it was terrifying. "Life is going to be boring. People will call me "Mr. Boring." But he was wrong. Unequivocally wrong. Life *before* was boring. It was the same routine, day in day out. Now, life is exciting and fresh in ways he never imagined. He claims his biggest problem in life now is a simple one; he wishes to live forever. To have longer to enjoy this newfound self and to experience more of what life has to offer without addiction standing in the way.

To return to the scenario I mentioned earlier in this chapter, was future Andrew to read this to his 30-year old self, I really don't know how he would take it. Of course, the benefits are a glorious thing. They paint nothing but positivity across the board, but for a man so blinded by his addiction, one who, especially at that age, didn't identify as having a problem, perhaps he would have been so naive to believe that the road he was already on could be just as good as the one his future self treads. But hindsight is a wonderful thing, and at the age of 55, Andrew can say with absolute certainty that he was wrong to ever believe such a thing. To think that a sober life was a boring life was foolish, ignorant and detrimental to himself and the people around him. When he made that fateful decision on February 27th 2018, he started life anew.

. . . .

Andrew recalls that, as a child, he couldn't listen to the song "I Wish it Could Be Christmas Everyday." He would listen to a lot of music in the front room, with his Mum and Dad and sister, Kath. George's favourite was Val Doonican's Greatest Hits. Songs such as Paddy McGinty's Goat, O'Rafferty's Motor

Car, Two Streets (which, ironically, has a metaphorical link to Andrew's story) would keep Andrew entertained on a regular basis, but when December rolled around and Kath whipped out her Wizard 45, Andrew would actually get teary-eyed, as he sat there really wishing it could be Christmas every day. And that was because George and Shirley worked very hard to make Christmas a very special time for Andrew and Kath. They may have been secondhand presents, or the financial value may not have been all that impressive, but they meant the world to young Andrew, who was so massively appreciative of the effort put in by his parents that he didn't want the experience to end. 25th December. Andrew would be awake at 3.30am, far too excited to sleep, where he would discover a pillowcase at the end of his bed stuffed full with presents. He'd jump straight out of bed and race through opening all his presents before Santa even had the time to arrive back at the North Pole. He'd then spend the whole day playing with his new toys and presents, seeing his wonderful family and generally having the best day. Christmas was the best.

However, when Andrew turned 18, Christmas took on a whole new form. Of course, he was still excited to receive and give gifts, but the excitement of a full day with his new best friend who he had become well acquainted with over the past half a year was even more exciting. So Christmas Day became another reason to drink, and drink to excess. But it was still a day that he loved greatly, drinking with friends and family. That was just what Christmas meant as he grew older. As the years continued on, Andrew started to think that Christmas could never be as good as when he was a child. But he was happy to discover he was wrong, once he met Christine. Christmas Day was then spent at her Dad's house, where all their family would be in attendance and the drink was flowing. They would play cards, smoke cigars, eat lots of food, laughing endlessly. Andrew quickly grew as excited about this new Christmas tradition as he was about his pillowcase as a child.

Christmas continued to change over the years as Chris and myself came along, where the excitement of watching us open our presents in the morning was the initial excitement, followed by a day of beer. So no matter what form it took, Andrew was a big fan of the Christmas period.

But after he turned 40, Andrew started to question what was happening to himself with regards to the festive season. Year after year, he started to enjoy Christmas less and less after a lifetime of loving it. For a while, he couldn't put his finger on it, but with that wonderful gift of hindsight he has since obtained, he can clearly identify the source of his dissatisfaction: Beer.

From his last day of work before the Christmas break until the day of going back, Andrew would overindulge like never before. So much so, that when it came to putting his overalls back on and getting back to it, they no longer fit. Not only that, but he had no money left, he was in a constantly hungover state and his anxiety was at an all-time high. And even though he knew things needed to change and that he needed to join in the country's tradition of drying out during January, he knew that he wouldn't. He knew that he couldn't resist continuing as he had been, piling on more weight and spending more money.

Speaking of money, it's a miracle that we managed to have the Christmas Days that we did. Whilst Christine was scrimping and saving every penny she could to make sure everyone got their presents and Christmas Day wasn't a wash out, Andrew was experiencing major beer fear, worried that he wouldn't have enough when the big day comes, making multiple trips to the supermarket to get more stocked up. The reason this induced fear in him was the notion of other people coming round to the house and drinking *his* beer, so he had to ensure he had enough to painfully hand over to others and to successfully intoxicate himself. The latter had a serious effect on the former, meaning Christine had a much lower budget to spend on presents and food. Eventually, this actual anxiety from Andrew's fear of the beer running dry made him resent people coming to our house on Christmas Day. "This is my beer, and nobody else's." As Christine (or Santa Claus) busily spent the Christmas Eve night laying out the presents for the morning, hoping to ensure myself and Chris had the best day possible, Andrew would be passed out on the sofa, snoring away loudly after a dosage that would make his basket look like a mere sample. The magic had died. Christmas was now soaked with the scent of alcohol. And though alcohol had played its part in the past during those days spent at Adrian and Margaret's house, it was now centre stage. Someone who has always shared in Andrew's passion for festivities is his old friend Jeff, who Andrew would speak to a lot during the Christmas period. He and Jeff would vent about how excited they were for the big day like giddy school children, but as the years went by and Andrew grew more bitter towards this time of year, he felt like he was lying to Jeff by joining in these conversations and feigning the same levels of excitement that Jeff was expressing. When he admitted to him that the excitement wasn't there anymore and that he didn't particularly enjoy

Christmas, it felt like he was insulting his best friend.

When Andrew faced down those fears on the day the beast arrived, Christmas played on his mind a lot. Perhaps the previous Christmas was still lingering for him, having been only two months prior, but as soon as he had put pen to paper and made his commitment, he doubted himself the ability to get through Christmas without drinking, but he pushed it to one side, thinking to cross that bridge when it arrives. But right through the year, especially in the months and weeks leading up to the 25th, it became the elephant in the room. He had made it through the best of the year: birthdays, holidays, gatherings, all without touching a drop and felt enormous pride for his achievement, as we all did for him, but Christmas was there, lingering in the corner of his mind, yelling at him phrases of doubt. He couldn't ignore his fear.

However, in the run up to Christmas 2018, Andrew's first as a sober man, he did things very differently. With his armoury of benefits outlined earlier, Andrew spent the weeks leading up to the day in ways no one could have anticipated a year earlier. He attended chapel services at the Kendal Unitarian Chapel, he partook of carol services at Kelbrook church and he and Christine accepted an invite from Snhoj to attend an evening where his partner would be singing with a group. Andrew invited his mother, Shirley along for the evening. Snhoj, in solidarity with his sober friend, didn't drink that night either, but they had a great evening, very cleverly adapting song lyrics to make them amusing to each other, the sort of thing that never really gets old, even with age. And while he could see people getting rounds of beers in, Andrew felt no envy, for the first time ever. During this evening, he realised Christmas had changed yet again and that he was really enjoying the festive mood with no liquid aids. Shirley loved it, Christine loved it and a great night was enjoyed by all. One that wouldn't have even been attended, had Andrew not given up the drink.

Christmas Day came, family came to our house to exchange gifts and have a laugh. Some of them drank, some of them didn't. Andrew had made sure enough alcohol was in the house to be able to offer visitors a drink, should they want one, but there was no fear there anymore, that they would be drinking his supply. That anxiety had gone. He enjoyed everybody's company throughout the day and retired to his bed at the end of it, having eaten too much food, but with a clear mind and a smile on his face, knowing that he would be waking up feeling as good as this. No hangover, no anxiety, no desperation to start drinking again.

Where he used to end the year feeling overweight, anxious, exhausted and hungover, starting the next year feeling as low as possible, he now ends it feeling positive and better than ever. But everything had hinged on that first sober Christmas. Had Andrew thrown the towel in there, caved and decided "it only happens once a year, might as well have a drink", this wagon would have come to a halt with the loss of a wheel, just as the rest had. Instead, it rolls ever onwards, with its driver eagerly anticipating the next Christmas, so he can get out to more carol services and enjoy the company of the people he loves, fully conscious and in the knowledge that when he puts the overalls back on, he won't need to squeeze into them, and his bank account won't be crying out in pain.

Chapter 12

If You Want the Rainbow, You've Got to Put Up With the Rain

"Do you know which "Philosopher" said that? Dolly Parton… And people say she's just a big pair of tits." - David Brent's wonderfully eloquent interpretation of Dolly Parton's immortal words. Whilst attempting to be anti-misogynistic, in typical Brent fashion, he falls into the trap of being misogynistic himself, but his heart was in the right place, by bringing Dolly's words to the people. And they're absolutely true. Unless you are somebody who sails through life with luck ever being on your side, if something is worth doing it, it more often than not comes with a degree of effort that can be off-putting, tiring and downright soul destroying at times. But once the end results are presented to you, the effort feels worth it. Pushing through that pain barrier, whether it be learning an instrument, sticking to a diet or, in this case, battling addiction, the rainbow is worth the rain. As humans, it is so easy for us to fold under the pressure of these trials and tribulations, to take shelter from the rain under the comfort of the known, like my Dad did each time he came off the wagon, but with the benefits I went at length to explain in the previous chapter now a part of his life, he knows that facing down said trials and winning out it in the end is the best outcome he could have hoped for.

Of course, it's easy now for my Dad to make that claim, since he has tasted the rewards at the end of the tunnel. For someone who has struggled to get past the pain barrier and is stuck firmly behind it, whether that is due to fear, reluctance, denial or myriad other reasons, they can only take these words at face value. It isn't until they're sat on that greener grass that they're mind frame can be altered, so to dismantle that barrier and reap the rewards takes will, determination and tremendous effort. Very rarely can such accomplishment be achieved overnight.

However, my Dad quickly learned that the effort does not cease, simply because you've reached your initial goal.

. . . .

Andrew weathered the storm. That Tuesday morning when he scrolled in his diary, the next chapter of his life began. The first week was tough, despite the encouraging words of Craig Beck and his wife, but as the following Tuesday rolled around, he took that same diary and wrote the number 1 on the top left of the page. He circled it, for extra clarity. Week 2 came and went. 3, 4, 5, 6 and onwards in the traditional format of numbers increasing one at a time. He always made sure to wait until the Tuesday to scribe in his diary. Even though he believed in himself, he didn't want to tempt fate by making the mark in the diary on the Sunday or the Monday. But, despite his trepidations, he started to realise that he was breezing through it. He wasn't craving booze and he was starting to have his first taste of those wonderful benefits. The weight started coming off, the anxiety started to vanish, the mood swings became less frequent. What was there to not love about this decision? Of course, there were challenging times (which, albeit, were less challenging than he anticipated, ala Christmas), but overall, as he numbered and circled each and every Tuesday that came and went, he found that he had passed each milestone with ease.

Week 52/one whole year - Andrew had achieved something which, those who knew him, had deemed entirely impossible. A whole year without booze. It really was something worth celebrating, which he did. A few weeks prior, Andrew had been in a card shop with Christine when he noticed a pattern in birthday cards. As soon as they reached the 18 and up bracket, Birthday cards had pictures of beer and wine and champagne on a vast majority of cards. "You're X years old! Celebrate with a drink!" was the general vibe he noticed. But all the cards from 1 - 17, naturally, didn't. So he made a request to his wife. He asked, tongue firmly in cheek, if she could present him with a "Happy 1st Birthday" card when February 27th rolled around. He specified that the card should have a badge with it that he could wear. Wanting to celebrate the milestone just as much as he did, Christine did just that. When the day came, Andrew opened his eyes, grabbed his diary, which he kept on his bedside table and excitedly inscribed upon February 27th 2019 "52", circling it more than once. Christine presented him with his card, to celebrate his first birthday as his new, improved self, complete with badge, which he lovingly adorned on his overalls. He went to work (yes, even on his *birthday*, rather than taking a week off to celebrate), where friends and colleagues alike congratulated him on this incredible achievement. That day, Andrew felt remarkable, recalling it as feeling as though he had done one of the best things of his life. The day came to a close, sealing in the history books Andrew's first year as a sober man.

When he made that fateful decision a year earlier, not knowing what the future held, and secretly doubting himself somewhat, he had decided that a year was the aim. If he could achieve a year of no drinking, he would have accomplished what he set out to. Not that he intended to crack open a can on day 366, rather that once that line had been crossed, he assumed that that was addiction defeated. But what he was soon to realise was that once an addict, always an addict.

As the Summer months approached, Andrew grew increasingly restless. He found he was becoming anxious again and was growing resentful and bitter towards everyday things and his friends and family. Depression would strike, without warning. He began to resent even his job and started to consider a new career path, maybe even going back to the car trade. In all, he was suffering from feelings and emotions he had suffered when he was drinking daily. He had no understanding of why this was happening. Further down the line and following a little research, Andrew would discover he was suffering from a condition called "Dry Drunk Syndrome." Dry Drunk, or DDS, as we shall call it going forward, can lead to resentment towards loved ones, depression, fear of relapse and general negative emotions with regards to one's own struggle with addiction. For Andrew and the people around him, his attitude was similar to that hungover, daytime Andrew we had known for years, and concern was growing that he could soon get in touch with Al. But not knowing what he was going through and unwilling to discuss the issues lead to more psychological trauma. Some people - who were perhaps less aware of the troubles Andrew had experienced as a result of his drinking - told him he was only torturing himself, and that he should just get himself a drink and be done with it, something he could do so easily, for that instant gratification. However, after a year of living through the benefits, he knew that doing so would only lead to more dark days, so he managed to resist. Still, the issues persisted.

After greatly struggling through the months of May and June and starting to question his own motivations for not drinking and what his new aim should be (what's Andrew gonna do next?), Andrew decided to open up to his cousin and close friend, Shaun. He told him that he felt restless after achieving his goal of a year and was contemplating giving into temptation. He described it to him as the same feeling as being on a diet. Getting to your goal weight is a huge achievement, but then it's very easy to say, "I've achieved that now, so I can eat what I want again." Fall into that trap, and before you know where you are, all the hard work and weathering the storm was for nothing, because you'll be right back where you started. For Andrew, this equates to, "well, I don't have financial worries anymore, can I drink again?" Thankfully for Andrew, Shaun rightly pointed out that he was ending the "honeymoon period", a term often used to describe the period of time shortly after entering a new relationship, where your attention and energy are focused entirely on that person, their happiness and wellbeing all the time. Eventually, as you settle into a new life and routine with that person, your attention wavers and the relationship becomes a part of everyday life. This isn't a bad thing, but it can lead to bad decisions, given that it is a new mindset, compared to the one you have experienced for the last so many months. This is what Andrew was facing, after his breakup with Al, a particularly challenging period for a man whose patience is limited at best and whose attention span is short, always looking for the next exciting thing. For the first 12 months, his focus was entirely on shunning Al. It was at the forefront of his mind throughout every day as he drew nearer and nearer to that initial goal of one year. With that milestone passed and sobriety settling into its everyday place in Andrew's life, it was no longer the new, exciting thing. He'd got bored of this toy and he wanted a new one.

With Shaun's revelation delivered and Andrew conducting his own research into what this meant for him, along with discovering the meaning behind DDS, Andrew was equipped to continue onwards in his new life. It would just take a few more words of encouragement to reignite the flame underneath him, which Shaun delivered: "what you've achieved is amazing" he said. "You have to keep going now. Once you're clear of the honeymoon period, you'll see the benefits again. It's not as easy as you thought it was going to be over a long period of time, because you've not done it before, and that's shocked you, but keep going." And so he did. He put up with this unforecast shower, against all odds. Once it had cleared and Andrew refocused his attention on the bountiful pleasantries now a part of his life, the yearning for new ventures evaporated. He went back to the North East coast with his wife and dogs, he exercised regularly, and he had a refreshed outlook on his career as a decorator of distinction. The rainbow, so to speak.

For a long time, Andrew has been enamoured with motivational speakers (partly the impetus to write this very book) and has looked to them for encouragement, especially during this entirely new phase of his life. On reflection, people such as Brian Tracy, David Goggins, Simon Sinek and Tony Robbins, to name but a few, are the embodiment of the wisdom imparted on Andrew by his cousin, Shaun. Whatever field they have succeeded in has been through an incredible amount of effort, dedication and hard work. The dawning realisation as he entered year two was that he would have to stay focused on his goal and that his recovery wouldn't happen without it. If he was to lose focus, should another spot of rain strike without warning, Andrew could easily give in to temptation. But he realises now that living a sober life is his *ultimate* goal. Not just for a year, or for two, but to remain that way for the rest of his life. When he was drinking and fantasising about a life in which he could afford luxury cars and big houses in the Mediterranean, he thought that was what he wanted, but with a clear mind and the gifts of life providing him with a renewed energy, he now sees these desires as hollow and fleeting in comparison to a life of health and happiness.

The grey moments do come, however. As recently as one month ago (at the time of writing), Andrew faced a challenging spell of cravings whilst on a short break in St. Andrew's, Scotland with Christine. They had arrived in the picturesque town for the first time on a beautiful, sunny, Friday afternoon after 5 - 6 hours of driving. They had explored the town somewhat before heading back to their lodgings. During this exploration, Andrew had seen people sitting outside bars, cafes and restaurants, once again being directed by Al to sip their drinks in sight of Andrew. The Truman Show continues. But this time, it didn't affect him. He had genuine feelings of happiness for the people relaxing with a drink in the sun, but also knowing that it would do no good for him to join them.

However, after a couple of hours at the guest house in which they were staying, the couple headed back into town to look for somewhere to eat. By now, the sun had vanished and a cold front had blown in. Andrew was feeling tired and hungry after a long day of driving and his blood sugar had dropped very low. Each restaurant they tried, they were turned away from as they were full and so the hunger continued to grow as the temperature dropped. All of a sudden, the pubs and bars Andrew could see now, with his blood sugar as low as it was and his mood rapidly deteriorating, were much more enticing. Al was stood close by, whispering words of encouragement, "Go on, Andrew. One sip is all it takes and you'll feel loads better." Andrew agreed, Al was right. The state he was currently in, he felt as though he could run up to the nearest person with a pint in their hand, snatch it off them and drink it down in one gulp. He expressed his concerns to Christine, telling her he was in trouble and he had to do something about it quickly, before he fell off his perpetually accelerating wagon. Soon after, they found a small, backstreet pizza restaurant, with barely anybody in, an oft worrying sign for an eating establishment. But with the conditions as they were and the options truly limited, they made their way inside and were shown quickly to a table. Still agitated and feeling restless, Andrew made his decision in record time and the food and drink arrived in the blink of an eye. The drink - a large glass of Diet Coke. One gulp later and the cravings were gone completely. The food was delicious, the restaurant had a wonderful, warm atmosphere and what could have been a night of disaster turned out to be a resoundingly pleasant evening. The previous hour of struggle had felt like a test, sent by Al himself to test Andrew's resolve. Had he given in there and then, it would have all been over. And for what? The benefits of conceding to the nagging voice of craving in his head are entirely limited. The benefits of sticking to his guns are endless and ever growing. And Andrew knows that when these moments come, which they inevitably will throughout the rest of his life, he only needs to compare and contrast the two versions of his existence to know which is the most beneficial.

What's Andrew gonna do next? He's going to continue to make this endeavour his single greatest accomplishment, the thing he has committed the most to. The best thing he's ever done.

Chapter 13

The Light at the End of the Tunnel

Knowing how to bring an end to this ongoing story is difficult. It's difficult for me to know how to end it, as someone who has read countless books and with a good understanding of what makes a good ending. However, it's even more difficult for a man who for which the end of a book is uncharted territory. He's opened and started numerous throughout his life - he clearly loves a good start to a book - but rarely has his bookmark travelled further than 15 pages or so. I remember being on holiday with him a couple of years ago in Northumberland. We had just paid a visit to my favourite bookshop, Barter Books in Alnwick. As usual, I left with a stack of books that I still to this day haven't finished reading, but, rather impressively, my Dad decided to buy a book also. We spent the afternoon back at the house we were staying in for the week. It felt like a strangely sophisticated afternoon - a rare treat when Andrew is your father, believe me - we all (myself, my partner Charlotte, my Mum and my Dad) sat quietly and read the books we had bought that day. I grew tired, so I closed my eyes whilst they all continued to read. I woke up on the sofa in the living room and everybody had gone to do something else. I picked up the book my Dad had been reading and made note of the fact the bookmark was 15 pages in. I was quite impressed. For someone who doesn't read and has the attention span of an excitable toddler to sit down and quietly make progress in a book is commendable. However, a few months later, I remember picking up the book again to see how far on he was now. I opened the book to find the bookmark still resting neatly between pages 15 and 16. "Oh well" I thought "he tried." A few more months later, I was telling this story to someone whilst my Dad was there when he admitted to me that he didn't even read those 15 pages. He got bored after two and put the bookmark in that position to make it appear as though he had read that much. If only his commitment to not drinking could be applied to his want to get to the end of a book. But anyway, back to finishing the book you're currently reading - as I've mentioned before, I could go on to describe stories of times when my Dad had too much to drink, made an arse of himself in front of friends and family and was full of regret and remorse the next day. I could chronicle each and every attempt made to get on the wagon, only for it to screech to a halt two days later. But for anyone who has lived through addiction, or has lived alongside it, these things won't serve as a revelation. They're simply the norm. Maybe you've never witnessed somebody in the states my Dad has been in or maybe you've seen much, much worse - that is beside the point. As a doctor once told my Dad, if you need to have a drink a day, even if it's just one, then that is an addiction. The same applies for eating addictions, gambling, drugs or any other form addiction can take, the issue remains the same, and the key to resolving that issue is finding the thing that works for you to break out of those constraints that dictate your life.

My Grandad George used to say, "the answer is not in the bottom of a glass." This was something that always stuck with my Dad. He may not have acted on that advice all the time, rather, he would do the opposite, searching there nightly for the solution to his problems, but this quote from his Dad was right and he knew it, whether he was conscious of it or not. As *my* Dad went on to learn, the answer lies within yourself. It might sound cliche or slightly new age to say so, but the answer is in your own experiences and motivations. Knowing that you have an issue is the key to applying those motivations towards achieving your goal.

As we set out at the beginning of this book, I made sure to explain to you, the reader, that this book isn't a step-by-step guide on how to handle addiction - those books exist - but rather this book's main aim is to serve as inspiration. I can only speak for myself, as the interpreter of this story, when I say that my Dad's story inspires me a great deal. I always find myself saying "well, if my Dad can give up drinking, I can do this." I've always wanted to write a book. I've always thought it would be incredible to hold in my hand a finished book that I created. But I've never done it in the past. Like my Dad's dismal attempts at reading one, writing one has been something that I have given up on in the early stages. But my Dad's story of triumph over adversity lit enough of a flame under me to actually want to see it completed. When he came to me with the idea for the second time, it struck a chord with me straight away. I've seen the transformation with my own eyes. My Dad is a different person now. Admittedly, he is *still* intensely irritating, singing stupid, improvised songs in the shower in the morning, loudly enough to pull me out of whatever it is I've been dreaming of. He still re-watches the same films and old TV shows whenever he gets the chance. Still does stupid voices and characters when I'm drinking a cup of tea, hoping to see me spray it everywhere in a fit of laughter. But through all those annoyances, and even during those times, his entire aura has changed to a man who I am happier to spend time with and to collaborate with and to someone who I am overjoyed to tell that I am proud of what he has achieved. Maybe I don't tell him that often enough - he's rarely being sensible enough for me to express it without being mocked for doing so - but I am endlessly proud. That first Christmas Day he spent sober, I felt apprehensive all day. As much as I didn't want him to, I thought he was going to crack. After spending my entire life seeing my Dad behave a certain way, giving in to temptation so easily, I really didn't have faith that he would make it through the day without a drink. I think I'd even discussed with my Mum the possibility of him not making it through, trying to diffuse an argument that may not even be on the cards. I believe I said something along the lines of "please don't be too hard on him if he has a drink." But as you well know, he didn't have a drink. But right up until he stood up from the sofa, overstuffed on turkey and chocolates and announced it was time for him to turn in, I didn't believe it. I couldn't believe it. It was miraculous. I gave him a few minutes and then snuck out of the living room and went upstairs to see him. I hugged him and I simply said, "well done." I didn't need to say what for. He just laughed and said back, "cheers, Yicks."

Something I recently admitted to my Dad was that I used to worry that my Mum would leave him. I had lots of friends growing up whose parents weren't together anymore. They'd go between their Mums and Dad's houses regularly. But I never understood this growing up. My parents would never split up! But when my Dad was at his worst, slurring his words, talking absolute drivel and wasting what little money we had, I'd see my Mum sitting quietly each night, waiting until he passed out on the sofa or on the floor, before she'd put something on the TV she actually wanted to watch and got an hour or two to herself and her thoughts. How those thoughts didn't lead her to the decision to leave my Dad is a mystery to me, but I certainly imagined that must be what she was thinking. And then my overactive imagination would feed on that, picturing what would happen to my Dad if my Mum left him. I pictured a filthy, squalor little flat. Takeaway boxes were stacked up on the side in the kitchen and the sink was full of unclean plates and cutlery which had accumulated over a few weeks ("they need to soak" he'd tell me). It goes without saying, but there'd be a lot of empty lager cans and the smell of red wine would be forever in the air. And there he was, slumped on the sofa, asleep, empty peanut packets around him, empty cans on the coffee table and Only Fools and Horses on the TV. "I think I'll stay at Mum's tonight" I'd say to myself, as I quietly made my way back to the front door.

They were unpleasant thoughts and I still feel for my Mum that she had to live through that period of their relationship for such a long time. But when I see them together now, tackling mountainous treks, going to the gym, eating healthy home cooked meals, even just watching the latest Netflix series together, I see the fantasy life my Mum imagined. Her slim, athletic, generous, humorous man has returned to her. She put up with the rain, and the rainbow came.

My Dad wishes that he gave up his addiction earlier. He wishes future Andrew did visit him with his almanac in hand to point him in the right direction. But he didn't. Instead, Al and his basket kept him in their cold, metallic, vice-like grip for as long as they could. But when the hold gave way, a new life began for my Dad. Like a colourblind person seeing the beauty of the world for the first time, he awoke a sober man. He can't live in regret that he didn't throw the towel in earlier, because regret will earn him nothing and will only hinder the clean, sober days that are ahead of him. Instead, he can relish in the fact that he now knows that when he wakes up at 5am to go for a power walk in the fresh, morning air, that that is as good as he will feel all day - and he feels absolutely incredible.

Frequently Asked Questions

"If I have seen further it is by standing on the
shoulders of giants" - Sir Isaac Newton

Committing to a decision with potentially life changing outcomes comes, naturally, with an abundance of questions. Those questions are best answered by the people who have lived through the experiences. It is only through their trials and tribulations that we can learn what works, what doesn't and what we need to know to make the all-important steps to change. As my Dad started to settle into the life of a sober man, he came to realise that a lot of people had questions for him, just as he had done for the going clean pioneers who came before him. But where my Dad sought the knowledge of people such as Craig Beck, with questions on how to end his addiction, the questions my Dad often face are of a different nature. He finds that people tend to question his motivations and the benefits of quitting, of which there are many. I suppose one of the key features of this book is to highlight how those benefits can drastically alter the life of a person who struggles with addiction and to inspire others to claim those benefits for themselves. Perhaps even you yourself still have questions after having read this story.

I prepared a series of questions for my Dad, some of which he has told me he is asked on a regular basis, and some I feel would serve as beneficial to people who have read this book. Whereas the usual process for committing my Dad's story to book form has been to use me as a medium, translating his often excitable, rambling stories into a cohesive narrative, we felt it would be important to hear the answers to said questions in an unfiltered, natural way. The questions weren't known to my Dad beforehand and the answers are his gut reaction - exactly how he would respond were you to ask these questions to his face.

. . . .

Jonny: To begin, I want to ask you a question I know you get asked often - are you still not drinking? What do you think when people ask you this question?

Andrew: Yeah, the most frequently asked question I get is this. I can almost tell the people that are going to ask me this question. I get a feeling that it's coming; here we go, "are you still not drinking?" and it's gone on now for just shy of 3 years, hasn't it, and I don't know if they're asking for my benefit or for theirs. But anyway, I'd love to say, "does it look like I'm still drinking?" or "does it look like I've given up?" but you can't say that because that's rude and naughty and very, very naughty (laughs).

The answer is, obviously, no I'm not. I'm dying to say something rude due to the amount of times I've been asked, but I'm also flattered, and I think "great, nice one, thank you very much for asking - but no, I'm still not drinking." It's quite a simple answer, really.

J: That question is often followed up with "do you feel better for it?"

A: Well, that's another one where I'm dying to say "no, I feel like shit. I've lost three stone in weight and I've got more money in the bank than I've ever had" (laughs). You see, I'm trying to be funny and clever here, but I'm clearly not. But the answer is yes, it's always yes and I'm absolutely delighted to tell people that yes, I feel ace, I'm on top form and things are great, so, yes, I feel great, thank you very much for asking.

J: What do you think people expect you to say when they ask a question of that nature?

A: That's a good question. That's a really good question and I'll tell you why I think it's a good question; when me and Lordy (*Andrew's close friend, Lincoln Lord*) were out walking the other day, we were talking about how, even your best mates want you to fail at stuff so that they can probably say to people "I saw Dick Dock (*a nickname for Andrew*) the other day. I told you he would fail with that giving up ale job." And it's quite a weird one, because they don't *really* want you to fail, but in a sense, they do. And also, if they like a drink themselves, and again, this book and these answers aren't meant to lecture anyone, you always wonder whether there's a little bit of a reaction like, "shit, is he still sober?"

J: Well, I suppose that could be an ego thing. It's almost affecting their ego that you've been so successful at this, whether they want to carry on drinking or not.

A: I've done it. I've been there myself. It's almost like, well, I play guitar, so I say to a mate "are you still playing guitar?" and they reply "yeah, I've just got back from touring America" and you're almost not happy for them and your ego is jealous and even though you are happy for them... It's a weird one. I mean, I'm a lot better now, I'm not as bitter and twisted as I was when I was drinking. But it is a good question and I think it all comes down to ego.

J: Another one I know people ask you; why don't you just have a drink?

A: I love this question. I absolutely love it. Simple answer: there's nothing in it for me. Nothing in it for me. I'd love to have a drink. I'd love a bottle of wine, a beer with a massive meal and indulge. I'd love to, but there's nothing in it for me, and I can say that knowing what I know now. And that's my favourite question of all time now. Because people who ask me, when I say that, I believe, they get it. Whoever they are, I believe when I say, "there's nothing in it for me", they think "flipping heck, he's right, there is nothing in it for him." There is nothing in it for me. Apart from satisfying the little chimp sat on my shoulder craving it and wanting me to have it and I'd just be feeding the chimp and not myself, I'd get nothing from it. So yeah, I love that question just to be able to say that.

J: Could you not just have a couple of drinks a week, maybe like, one or two at a weekend? Because maybe when you made the decision to quit, you could have just weaned down to a couple a week rather than every night, so why did it have to be all or nothing?

A: Good question, again. And I think that is - when I was listening to Craig Beck's book (*Alcohol Lied to Me*), that book put it clearly to me that you can't do that. We've all tried that. And I was almost disappointed that Craig Beck's book told me that and pointed out to me that that doesn't work. I was waiting for it to pop up and say to me, "oh but, you know, to be fair, you like your ale don't ya, you like a glass of wine and a beer... seems a shame... if you think you're capable, just treat yourself every now and then," but that didn't happen. It made it clear that, sadly for me, that wasn't an option. I answered all the questions in Craig's book about whether I was in fact a social drinker or whether I was addicted to the stuff. Once I answered all the questions, I knew what I already knew, so it had to be a full stop. And now that I am where I am, I'm glad that it was a full stop.

J: It's stated in the book that your main inspiration for quitting at first was your financial situation, yet when you faced eviction from your house and was made bankrupt, why didn't you quit there and then?

A: Because that *was* the basketful of happiness. That was the only thing I had left at that point. That was the thing that made me even more selfish than I already were. That was the epitome of Christmas every day, I'm allowed to do this, have you seen what's happened to me? I'm a victim in all this. So, give me some money, because I want an ale. Whoever you are, just give me some money. That was what made me more selfish and bitter about everything. That was absolutely my way of saying, "bollocks to everything, I'm having an ale." It was my own gratification after everything I'd been through.

J: How often do people tell you that you didn't have a problem to begin with?

A: It doesn't happen so much now, but at the beginning, with family members and friends and what have you… It was something I noticed when I tried going to AA and stuff, I got the feeling that it was a case of "my uncle is bigger than your uncle, my car is faster than your car" type situation - all this sort of malarkey. That comes into everything. Even when people have got serious issues going on, the reason people could ask that question is because people didn't see me sat outside a library at 11am supping a bottle of Diamond White or whatever, so therefore, you know, it comes back to people thinking well he drinks premium lager and expensive wine, so he hasn't got a drink problem, that's someone who enjoys a nice drink.

J: So, do you think you were good at hiding it? Was that your intention; to make people think you didn't have a problem?

A: No, because I was proud of being a drinker, I thought I was great. I told people from a young age - you know, back in the early chapters where I said I wanted to be a drinker - I wasn't hiding anything. I wanted to be known as a big drinker and a "top banana" you know, a party animal, where when I walk in people go "wahey, here he is look", so, no, I didn't want to hide it.

J: But what about towards the end, where there were none of that; people admiring you and thinking you're a legend, you were just sat, on your own, in the same seat supping ale all night every night? Did you still have pride in your abilities then?

A: No. No no no. That's a really good question, that.

J: So, I suppose it changed over time then?

A: Well, my last birthday drink, when I was 52, when I went to the Craven Heifer. Richard Wilson (*Andrew's lifelong friend and godfather to Chris*) still laughs about it to this day, when Olivia was there (*Chris's partner*) and Chris - you didn't go to that, did you? No, I wondered why we'd had such a good time, you weren't there - so Olivia got up to go, and I was "arseholed" - I'm talking utterly out of it - and I went (in some strange, pseudo-impression of Austin Powers) "are you going now baby?" and Richard Wilson absolutely howled and our Chris looked at me and went, *"what?!"* and I remember laughing my head off thinking that was funny and Chris (*who lived in Kelbrook at the time and so the Craven Heifer was his local*) was well embarrassed and was telling me he had a reputation to uphold and what have you. But, on the way home, I was desperate for some more ale, because obviously I was only pissed out of my head at that point, I needed to get shitfaced to the point of passing out on the floor on that particular Tuesday night (said with sarcasm, of course). And Chris videoed me in the car, shouting at your Mum telling her, "get to Rolls Club on the way back, we can get in for last orders," and your Mum were effing and blinding at me and I was saying, "what's up with you, it's my birthday," you know, justifying like I did at that time, as a selfish drunk. Anyway, we didn't go to the club and me and your Mum fell out about that because it was *my* birthday and *I* say what we're doing - you know. And I've seen that video since and, my God, that is the most cringing thing I've ever seen of myself. Arguing with your

Mum because I wanted a drink. And Chris was laughing, but I wasn't, and neither was your Mum.

I don't know if that answers the question or if I'm just waffling, but it did change, and I did become embarrassed.

J: It's funny because, you say you cringed looking at this video of Chris's, but the amount of moments that reside in my head where I saw you acting a fool after a drink are endless. It changed you every time. I remember coming back from a meal once and it was Chris's birthday and he was sat in the front of the car playing Beatles CD's and you were sat in the back, very drunk saying, "they're fucking shit. Ahh, turn this shit off, bloody well shit this band, get that off." I just tried to ignore you because I knew you didn't even think that, you were just being bitter because we'd left the restaurant where the food and drink was.

A: How mad is that, since they're one of my all-time favourite bands (laughs). I must have only been doing that to annoy Chris and because I was bitter. I'm sorry, that's awful (laughs). But yeah, people didn't know I had a problem, despite that. They just thought that I liked a laugh and that's who I was. They just didn't realise. Lads at work would ask me how much I'd had to drink the night before and they were impressed.

J: I suppose it's like how I said in the intro that when I was young, I didn't know you had a problem, I just thought that all Dads drink and it wasn't until I got older that I realised that they don't, or at least, not to that extent.

A: All I know is I had a big enough problem that it very nearly cost me everything I'd worked my whole life to own, so yeah, I think it's safe to say I had a problem.

J: Moving on, when cravings set in and you feel like you really need a drink, what's your main inspiration - the main thing you think of to stop yourself from giving in? Is it different each time?

A: I always come back to there being nothing in it for me. It's that answer every time. It might hurt and be painful at the time, you know, I might be driving home from work and I'm tired and my blood sugar levels are low, and I've had a brilliant week which I'd like to celebrate, and I start thinking of people who I know will be having an ale tonight. And I go past pubs and I see people standing there having a beer and it gets me. It really gets me. But then I just remember, there's nothing in it for me. And I'm happy for the people who are ordering ale and I'm happy for the people sitting at home having a gin and tonic before their tea - I'm delighted for them and I think that helps me too. I am genuinely happy for *anyone* who gets enjoyment out of a drink, but I just know that there is nothing in it for me, not anymore. I've realised that after all this time. And that's how I cure my cravings.

When I gave up drinking, at the start, for my own vanity, I told myself that if anybody asked me whether quitting was easy, I would tell them yes. I thought, I've got to tell them yes, because otherwise people will think "well why are you even bothering then?" If I tell someone that it's *unbelievably* easy to give up drinking, it would be a lie. I could tell them about the benefits I've come to understand since giving up, but to say it was easy to begin with would be a lie. It's like, if I saw a body builder who's worked incredibly hard to look the way they do and I say to them "you look amazing, is it easy?" well, no, of course it isn't. You need to go to the gym every single day, stick to a very restricted diet and work very hard - but the results are obvious. And knowing that now, if somebody asks me if it's easy *now*, I'll tell them the truth, that it isn't. And if they say, "well what the bloody hell have you given up for then?" it's because I know that I'm better in every way without it.

J: I think that was something you worried about when we were preparing for the "rainbow" chapter. You were worried that if we said to people that just as things are starting to look good again, after all the benefits we'd outlined, that things could easily go wrong again and that that could put people off. Is that fair to say?

A: Yes, I was worried. I was worried, but I'm not anymore. Because imagine Wayne Tancock (*owner of Intershape Gym, where Andrew trains*) saying, "well... I'm going to have to be honest with you... this weight training business, to get to look how I do, erm... you're going to have to train as hard as I have getting up at 6 o'clock every morning to train 365 days a year... I'm sorry if that's put you off." Well, if you want to look like Wayne, you're going to have to do what Wayne's done. That's why I use people like that as a bit of a focus because, if you want to look like that, you need to put in the effort and it's the same with this. It's all about consistency, and his has clearly paid off.

J: I know that your intentions throughout this whole book has been to never lecture on the subject of addiction - whether that's alcohol, drugs or whatever that may be. But would you try to interfere and help a friend and try to

redirect their life if things appeared to be getting out of hand for them in terms of addiction?

A: If I didn't say yes to that, I'd sound out of order, wouldn't I? But I might have a cunning plan to get them to talk about it, knowing what I know now. Maybe I'd go straight in and give them a load of stick and abuse, having a joke with them - call them "pissy no ho" (*as in, pissed up no hoper, a nickname my Dad picked up*) and say things like "can you see straight today", the kind of jokes people use to say to me. Snhoj used to call me "piss brain" when we were at work, sarcastically saying that my drink the night before will help with my decorating that day. I had that every day, so there was no escaping it. Or maybe I'd be more direct and just go up and say, "sorry to ask, please don't think I'm a bigheaded sod because I don't do it anymore, but is this bugger [addiction] getting on top of you? I maybe wouldn't say directly "have *you* got a problem?" I would say is *it* getting you. You know, maybe turning it round, to say that addiction has got you, rather than accusing them of getting *it*. I know that's what happened with me, it got me.

I feel like I'm waffling a bit there again, but I remember a friend who had a serious drink problem, and they were asking me for advice. This is only recently, and they said they knew that I'd given up and they were saying, "I don't know what to do, Andrew." I said to them, "do you know what would be a good thing to do? Get the empty bottle and put them on a shelf and maybe somebody like your partner talking to the bottles and yourself and saying, "now what have you been doing to him? You've made him into a pisshead, haven't you? You've been making him drink you again, haven't you?" and, you know, just have a bit of a laugh with it and direct the lecture towards the bottles, rather than to the poor sod who has been taken over by this. Of course, there's a very serious side to it, but let's not be too serious here, because there is enough of that going on.

J: You've responded numerous times throughout these questions with "what's in it for me?" but what would you say to someone who asked *you* that very question, if they were considering quitting?

A: It depends on their circumstances. Say they were going around in a battered old Ford Fiesta worth about £30 - like I was doing - and they can't afford the MOT because that means they can't then buy a drink - a good, highly qualified decorator, earning good money an hour, but you can't even afford a van because all the money you earn is going on the drink - and you're making yourself look a prat day in day out, it's clearly obvious what's in it for them to give up. But it depends how much I know about a person's situation, you know, I might tell someone who was in a situation like that that I now go on 3 - 4 holidays a year. Not to show off, but to say well that's what's in it for you. I might use examples like that one. Say, for argument's sake, when I was drinking all the time, I played golf a bit, but I couldn't really afford to, because my priorities were the ale. So Ghyll Golf Club costs about 5/600 quid a year. Colne Golf Club, same again. Nelson Private Golf Club, about a grand a year. So, if somebody had said to me, "why don't you join Ghyll Golf Club then?" I'd have simply told them that it's too dear. But if you'd said to me "why don't you join Ghyll, Colne *and* Nelson - all three, take your pick which one you go to, *and* save three grand a year" and I'd say, well, what do I have to do to do that? And they say "quit drinking" - what, so you're telling me all I have to do is quit drinking and I can join all three and still save a further three grand on top of that? Bang on. If you commit the amount of money you're spending on ale on a yearly basis to that hobby, that is what you can afford for yourself, plus £3,000 - £4,000 saved on top. Simple as that. I know that if somebody had said that to me once I acknowledged I had a problem and that I wanted to quit, that would sink into my head and I'd think "wow."

So that's a specific example for me, but I'd just try and explain the benefits like that. And I wouldn't be making anything up, it's just the truth. Because the truth really is unbelievable. It really is. But again, I would never tell them, "you shouldn't be drinking," because that isn't the way to do it.

J: Do you wish you'd quit earlier?

A: Great question. With hindsight, if I'd been sober when I was, say, 30, when I'd just started working at Preston's [BMW] and I'd been able to stay focused on my career - where I was popular, even with the people at BMW Great Britain, who knows where I'd have been? But I wasn't focused on my job, and I realise that now. Consistency needed to come into play. But my consistency was, and always has been, focused on ale. So yes, I do wish I'd quit earlier, but like your Mum said to me, you can't think like that, because you are where you are now due to your choices. Who knows how things would have worked out differently?

Do I wish I'd quit when I was 18? Who knows where that would have taken me? As Val Doonican once said (starts singing), "two streets, which one will I take? If I take the first one, I'll be on my own" (laughs). I never understood that song, but I do now (laughs).

J: What would you say is your best piece of advice for someone who is considering quitting?

A: I can only say what worked for me: listen to Craig Beck's audiobook, Alcohol Lied to Me. Because that worked for me. It spoke to me. I actually once emailed Craig and I told him how that book was literally aimed at me. He was a man in business and with ambitions and alcohol took him, so I felt like me and him had the exact same problem. And once I heard it coming from him - on the very first day I started listening to that book, I thought to myself "I want to do that. I want to help people; I want to do that." I know that that is typical of me, running before I walk. I hadn't even been sober for more than 3 hours and I wanted my own book on quitting drinking. Genuinely, I found it that inspiring. I knew in those first couple of hours that Craig Beck was going to help me. I just knew it.

I'm not saying that will work for everyone, there's a lot of options out there for somebody who wants to quit. But that's what worked for me, 100%.

J: Finally, what is your ultimate goal?

A: Stay sober. Own a Ferrari? No, no. A house in Majorca? That used to be my goal. But no, stay sober. As Brian Tracy says, you need daily goals, and I only have one daily goal: stay sober. If I stick to that, one day, I may have a Ferrari, or a house in Majorca. Those things don't interest me as much anymore, but it becomes possible. I know for a fact that everything I want and wish for can be obtained eventually as long as I stick to that ultimate goal.

Epilogue

AI always be by your side!

I first met Andrew in Kelbrook in 1982. I had called into a small pub called "The Craven Heifer", to see who was already embracing the good word of the drinking bible and who perhaps was yet to sip upon the hallowed nectar. I glanced around the bar, taking in the sweet sight of the locals throwing down pint after pint of the amber fluid when I noticed a young man, sat in the corner with a glass of Coke in his hand, admiringly watching the men. I could sense straight away that he longed for a taste of the good stuff, that the Coke was merely a substitute for what he could not legally obtain. I quietly approached him, taking my place by his side. I leant forward, closely in at his ear and quietly explained that his time would soon come, and that when it did, our relationship would blossom. I could feel an instant bond between the two of us, as though he was desperate for me to be a part of his life. I stood up from the table, gave him one more quick glance and left the pub. But I would return, when my new friend was old enough to embrace all that I stand for.

One year later, I found myself, once again, in the Heifer. I'm not sure what it was, but I felt a calling from this place on this evening, like I was destined to revisit and at this very time. As I walked through the front door, my thinking was confirmed, as I saw the young man from last year, holding in his hand a shot of rum. I was delighted to see that he was moments away from his first step towards enlightenment. I quietly moved closer, to get a good view of his baptismal moment, keeping enough distance as to not add pressure. The liquid went down in one throw back of his head. That was the moment. The moment that introduced me to someone I would hold very dear in my life. He would come to me on any occasion. We would celebrate together, we would be sad together, we'd party when others had kaffled and we'd hide away from the world together, lost in a realm of distorted vision, nonsensical thoughts, standing atop a steeple of our creation. We felt happier in each other's presence and we made each other feel untouchable. Nothing could penetrate the walls we built around us when we spent time together. And when we weren't in each other's company, I could feel him longing for me, wishing the time away until we would be together again.

In reality, I had him wrapped around my little finger. From that first taste at the age of 18, I became a part of him. Sometimes, I would hear him wake up in a morning and exclaim that he wasn't going to see me that day, that he'd had enough of me. The cheek of it! How dare he say such a thing? He'd start out his day with a sense of defiance and I'd hear him repeatedly make his claim, to his wife, his children, his colleagues... but it would never take long for me to apply the pressure. I knew him inside out. I knew exactly which buttons to press and at what times. I could set my watch by the regularity of his turn around, as he came crawling back to me at the end of a working day. We would merrily trawl through the shelves of the local petrol station shop, picking up cans of lager, strong, red wine and all sorts of assaulting snacks. I would see the happiness emitting from his very soul. Knowing what he had sitting in his basket and the incredible bliss that it would provide, once he got home, slouched on his sofa. It changed the way Andrew behaved. This was the Andrew that I wanted to be around, as often as possible.

In the early days of our relationship, he could see no downside to spending time with me. A lot of people I encounter, I may only be acquainted with briefly, as the aftertaste I leave can be enough to scare some people away. When they say, "never again", sometimes, they mean it, or we won't have a catch up for a while. Others, it may only be a week or so before we're back in the nightclub again, drowning the night away. Young Andrew, on the other hand, would awaken feeling fresh and excited about when we could next party together. These are the kind of friends I like. The ones who don't turn their back on me, just because I come with some undesirable side effects.

However, as Andrew started to get older, he started to point the finger at me increasingly often. He would blame me for his weight gain, his high blood pressure, his headaches, his anxieties, for the fact his latest bike ride felt like a real struggle. This is when he would start telling people we were going our separate ways. I think he even managed to convince himself, in the wee hours of the morning, when he would awaken with a thick head and feeling nauseous. But, as I already explained, it wouldn't take long for him to come to me with his tail between his legs, stating that really, he just wanted to spend time with me. It didn't matter that he would appear as a walking contradiction to everyone else. The happiness I provided to him was enough to leave him blind to everything else. As we sat in his living room together, nightly, his wife looking for anything else to do, his sons away in their rooms, he would tell me how better things were when we were together, digging deeper and deeper into the sandpit, until it was deep enough for us to submerge him in it entirely.

We shared many happy times together, throughout the years, and I know for a fact that Andrew looks back on some of them favourably now. I mean, who could forget that first holiday we went on, with his friends? We had such an incredible time together, all of us, and only happy memories remain of then. The same can be said of many occasions we were together! Don't forget, I was by his side when him and Christine first got together. I was there through birthdays, Christmas's, holidays, just about every special occasion. I sat idly by while he was out of work with his back condition, ready and waiting with a cold can of Stella.

I was well aware of the financial trouble Andrew was facing at one point, and I knew it was down to the time he'd been spending with me, but, as I say, our time together was too precious for me to care for the consequences, and Andrew definitely saw me as an escape rope from everything that was bad. So, I would continue to apply the pressure on him, until he came calling for me in the evening, and I would never fail to bring him out of his stupor and into a state of temporary euphoria.

Then, one day, everything changed. A few years ago, there came a day where Andrew didn't come and meet me at the petrol station for his usual basket of supplies. I'd heard him discuss with Christine that day that he was giving me up, that he would never see me again. But I'd heard all that talk before, countless times. In fact, there'd even been times when we wouldn't see each other for a few weeks, maybe even a month or two, sometimes. The weather had been very bad that day, the roads were covered in thick layers of snow. I thought briefly that perhaps he had just decided to not brave driving down to the garage that day, but a bit of snow had never come between us before. Something felt off. I thought back over the day, to the times I had attempted to call out to him, as I always did. He hadn't been at work, due to the weather, but he had spent the majority of the day with some earphones in. I don't know what he was listening to, but I wonder now whether this was the trigger for his change in behaviour? I tried not to overthink things, put the day aside as a temporary blip and went up into town to see if there was anybody else I could bring under my wing.

The next day, I made numerous attempts to contact Andrew. At times, it seemed he may be coming around to the idea of seeing me that evening. I could see cracks forming and my confidence came racing back, only to be shattered once again, when he stood me up for the second day running. I was furious. Over the course of a week or two, I applied so much pressure to Andrew that he felt perpetually ill. This was usually a surefire method to bring Andrew back to the fold, as he was a believer of the old adage, "the hair of the dog", a phrase that has saved uncountable relationships of mine. So, I would continue to lather on negativity: headaches, anxiety, a constant feeling of needing to throw up; I wasn't going to let Andrew go without a fight. But still, he continued to avoid me. *Me*, one of his oldest, closest friends. How many times had I been there for him when things looked bad? Ok, I was a bit manipulative at times, but even he admits how happy I made him on a daily basis! I was a guarantee for him. A surefire way to make things better. Yes, I bankrupted him, but he doesn't need anything else! As long as he has me!

It's been years now, and me and Andrew have still not been reacquainted. There have been occasional times when I have attempted my old methods of applying pressure, to see if I can possibly tempt him to come and see me. I could feel him considering the possibility of an evening with me, could hear his thoughts, as he tried to justify to himself that he could maybe just have a drink or two. Why not? Everyone else does it! Why shouldn't he. I would be all but rubbing my hands in anticipation, when, as quickly as the thought had entered his mind, it had vanished, leaving him with nothing but feelings of triumph, as he shunned me once again.

Unfortunately, I feel it may be time for me to admit that myself and Andrew shall never have the relationship we once had. I see him from time to time, when I'm spending time with other friends of mine, sipping away at his lime and soda, completely ignoring me. I barely recognise him anymore. It blows my mind to think how much he used to depend on me. How much he would rely on me as his ultimate source of happiness. I supplied him with a daily flow of fuel. His body functioned in the way it did because of what I provided for him. I changed his life. I was his best friend.

Acknowledgements

Andrew would like to thank

First and foremost, I need to thank Craig Beck. If I hadn't discovered his book in the first place, this book wouldn't exist. Kendal Unitarian Chapel played an important part in my development, as I tried to add value to myself - and they continue to do so. But most importantly, I want to thank my wife and family for sticking by me while I was in the worst place. I also have to thank Jonny, of course, for his bit of a contribution... A massive thank you to Robert Lee for designing the book cover - someone who I have a massive amount of respect for since I've loved Pulled Apart By Horses for so long. It feels great to have him on board. A huge thank you to Tiiu Shelley for proof reading the book, to Paul Mason, Matt Heap, Shaun O'Neill and Mike Warburton for being our "test readers" and giving us their thoughts. I'd also like to thank all the friends and family who helped us, either financially or with kind words over the years. You likely don't realise just how much of a problem I had and just how much you assisted. Alos, a huge heartfelt thank you to Mr & Mrs R who if it wasn't for their generosity and kindness, we wouldn't be where we are today.

Jonny would like to thank

I have to first thank my Dad, for showing me that I actually had it in me to finish writing a book. His continued encouragement, especially when I was doubting my own writing was what made me carry on and not throw in the towel. I'm also massively inspired by his story, in that it proves I can achieve anything. This same thanks to my Mum, who contributed as much as anybody else, present at all book "meetings" and discussions, as well as writing her own brilliant chapter. Thank you to my partner, Charby and her family for all their support and encouragement in everything I do. Thanks to my brother, Chris, for his contribution, even if it was slightly painful to get it out of him. Thanks to my Honeyspider band mates, Matt, Paddy and Tom, for giving me a chance to escape writing for a little while to work on music. Enormous thank you to Rob for reaching out and offering to do the cover design - something I really did not expect! Everybody listen to Pulled Apart By Horses, they're the best! Thank you to Tiiu Shelley for generously proof reading and pointing out the hundreds of errors I made throughout - I think I need to go study English a bit more. Thank you to Matt, Mike, Paul and Shaun for their feedback, also. It was really nice to hear you say nice things about something I have spent so much time on. Thanks to all my friends who have asked me how I am getting on with writing - I'm actually a little bit overwhelmed just how many people have continued to check in over the past year - you know who you are. Thank you to my pups, Moby and Lulu for being the best animals in the World. And lastly, thank you to everyone reading this now. It blows my mind to think that you have picked up this book, shown an interest in my Dad and my family and made it to this point. My appreciation is endless.

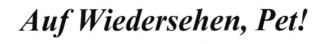

Auf Wiedersehen, Pet!

Printed in Great Britain
by Amazon

58069123R00159